D0809564

Ethical problems in clinical practice

To the memory of Ove Damborg Holm,
a good man and a wonderful father

Ethical problems in clinical practice

The ethical reasoning
of health care professionals

Søren Holm

Manchester University Press

MANCHESTER and NEW YORK

distributed exclusively in the USA by ST. MARTIN'S PRESS

174.2
H 73e

Published by Manchester University Press
Oxford Road, Manchester M13 9NR, UK
and Room 400, 175 Fifth Avenue, New York, NY 10010, USA

Distributed exclusively in the USA by
St. Martin's Press, Inc., 175 Fifth Avenue, New York,
NY 10010, USA

Distributed exclusively in Canada by
UBC Press, University of British Columbia, 6344 Memorial Road,
Vancouver, BC, Canada V6T 1Z2

British Library Cataloguing-in-Publication Data
A catalogue record for this book is available from the British Library

Library of Congress Cataloging-in-Publication Data
Holm, Søren.
    Ethical problems in clinical practice : the ethical reasoning of
health care professionals / Søren Holm.
        p.   cm.
    Includes index.
    ISBN 0–7190–5049–9 (cloth).—ISBN 0–7190–5050–2 (paperback)
    1. Medical ethics.   2. Clinical medicine—Decision making.
I. Title.
    [DNLM: 1. Ethics, Medical.   W 50 H747e 1997]
R724.H59   1997
174'.2—dc21
DNLM/DLC   97–13570

ISBN 0 7190 5049 9 *hardback*
      0 7190 5050 2 *paperback*

First published 1997
01 00 99 98 97   10 9 8 7 6 5 4 3 2 1

Typeset in Walbaum
by Northern Phototypesetting Co. Ltd, Bolton
Printed in Great Britain
by Bell & Bain Limited, Glasgow

Contents

Our discussion will be adequate if it has as much clearness as the subject-matter admits of; for precision is not to be sought for alike in all discussions, any more than in all the products of the crafts. Now fine and just actions, which political science investigates, exhibits much variety and fluctuation, so that they may be thought to exist only by convention, and not by nature. And goods also exhibit a similar fluctuation because they bring harm to many people; for before now men have been undone by reason of their wealth, and others by reason of their courage. We must be content, then, in speaking of such subjects and with such premises to indicate the truth roughly and in outline, and in speaking about things which are only for the most part true and with premises of the same kind to reach conclusions that are no better. In the same spirit, therefore, should each of our statements be *received*; for it is the mark of an educated man to look for precision in each class of things just so far as the nature of the subject admits; it is evidently equally foolish to accept probable reasoning from a mathematician and to demand from a rhetorician demonstrative proofs.

Aristotle. Nicomachean Ethics, Book 1, ch. 3, 1094b–1095a. In: Ackrill J. L. (ed.), *A New Aristotle Reader*. Oxford: Oxford University Press, 1987: p.364.

Preface

> And further, by these, my son, be admonished: of making many
> books there is no end; and much study is a weariness of the flesh.
> (Ecclesiastes 12: 12)

The topic of the book you hold in your hand is the ethical reasoning of health care professionals. How do they identify ethical problems, and how do they think about these problems
when they have identified them? The book is also about the
use of empirical studies in health care ethics, especially studies using qualitative research methodology.

In deference to the tradition in the health sciences, the
style of the writing is 'realist'. The history and sociology of science shows us that the actual research process is often much
more messy than the sanitised descriptions presented in published research papers, and there may be good reasons to
change to a more 'confessional' style [1]. I have resisted this
temptation, but the reader should be aware that a realist tale
always presents a rationalised version of the research process,
leaving out much of the detail about the more practical problems in research, problems that present scientific standards see
as irrelevant but which nevertheless influence both process and
outcome. I have, however, tried to leave in a description of as
many of these problems as can be accommodated within a
realist style of writing.

I am not a literary writer; and although I can see some

merit in a literary and rhetorical approach to writing in the
social sciences [2], I still think that what is primarily important is the message and not the style. In some places this belief
has prompted me to choose clarity in meaning at the expense
of grace of expression.

With regard to the content I have tried to heed the advice
given by Aristotle and Edgar Allan Poe in the two quotations
at the beginning and end of this book. In empirical research
there is a great temptation to seek greater clarity than the subject-matter admits of, but I have tried to resist this temptation,
and to make it clear that I do, for the most part, only 'indicate
the truth roughly and in outline'.

I hope that the reader will also remember that 'it is the
mark of an educated man to look for precision in each class of
things just so far as the nature of the subject admits'. There is
no reason to believe that we will ever be able to gain the same
clarity in our analyses of the moral reasoning of actual human
beings as we are able to gain in our theoretical analysis of
moral philosophy. The human mind is infinitely complex. Its
workings may be beyond computability [3], and this complex-
ity seems to spill over into moral reasoning.

If readers remember this caveat, there is also a good
chance that they will be able to keep their own version of 'The
summer dream beneath the tamarind tree', and continue to be
appropriately sceptical towards this, or any other, attempt to
say the last word about moral reasoning.

This book is written in English, although all the empirical
research was done in Denmark, and all interviews were conducted in Danish. The main drawback of this is that the report
on the qualitative analysis is in a different language from the
one in which the study was conducted. Great care has been
taken in translation, both of the analytical categories and of
the interview quotes presented. The translation has not always
been easy. Spoken Danish, like most other spoken languages,
has a much looser structure than its written counterpart. I have
tried to retain this 'oral' feeling in the translation.

I have used the terms medical ethics, biomedical ethics,

health care ethics, and bioethics interchangeably. When I use medical ethics, it is therefore in a broader sense than 'doctors' ethics', and when I use bioethics it is in a narrower sense than 'ethics concerned with living beings'. This use of the terms is consistent with that used in the Office of Technology Assessment background paper *Biomedical Ethics in U.S. Public Policy*, which states:

> With time, however, bioethics has become synonymous with biomedical ethics. *This report uses bioethics and biomedical ethics interchangeably, excluding areas of inquiry that others might include (e.g. environmental implications or the use of animals in experimentation).* [4, p. 2, emphasis in original]

I also use the words 'ethical' and 'moral' as synonyms. I am fully aware that it is possible to make the distinction between 'ethical' and 'ethics' for theoretical considerations and 'moral' and 'morality' for the rules flowing from the considerations or transmitted through tradition. I do not think that this distinction is very firm in everyday language, and I see no advantage in using it as a stipulative technical distinction.

References

1 Van Maanen, J., *Tales of the Field – On Writing Ethnography*. Chicago: The University of Chicago Press, 1988.

2 Richardson, L., *Writing Strategies – Reaching Diverse Audiences*. Sage University Paper Series on Qualitative Research Methods (vol. 21). Beverly Hills, CA: Sage, 1990.

3 Penrose, R., *Shadows of the Mind: A search for the Missing Science of Consciousness*. Oxford: Oxford University Press, 1994.

4 US Congress, Office of Technology Assessment. *Biomedical Ethics in U.S. Public Policy* (background paper). Washington, DC: US Government Printing Office, 1993.

Acknowledgements

This book is the result of a project that has received economic support from several sources. Personally, I have been the recipient of a research fellowship from the Faculty of Health Sciences, University of Copenhagen. The Danish Research Academy and Christian og Ottilia Brorsons Rejselegat for Yngre Videnskabsmænd have supported me during two visits to research centres abroad, and grants from Fonden af 1870, Direktør Jacob Madsen og Hustru Olga Madsens Fond, Anna og Jakob Jakobsens Legat, Lægeforeningens Forskningsfond, and Vibeke Binder og Povl Riis' Fond have made various parts of the research possible.

Many people have contributed to the book through discussion and comment. I cannot thank them all here, but I would like to mention my colleagues Henrik Wulff, Povl Riis, Peter Rossel, Michael Norup, and Klemens Kappel.

The two secretaries at our department, Kirsten Kjær and Hanne Christensen, have contributed to this work in many ways both directly through their work, and indirectly by contributing to the excellent working environment at the department.

I also want to thank all the doctors and nurses who have given generously of their time and insights during the interviews.

Last, but not least, I want to thank the one person without whom the project and this book would not have been completed: Hanne Krogh Krüger, who with great efficiency and skill transcribed all the interview tapes.

1

Introduction

The initial question

The purpose of the empirical study and theoretical analysis presented in this book is to try to understand how health care professionals reason about ethical issues, and how the organisation of health care influences clinical decisions with an ethical component. My reasons for choosing this research topic and methodology are partly my interest in philosophical health care ethics, and partly my own experiences as house officer in two departments in a large regional hospital and as a teacher of medical ethics.

The present state of medical ethics

Medical ethics, or bioethics, is a relatively new academic subject which began to expand during the late 1960s. Several scandals in medical research, including the occasion when a Seattle 'God committee' chose candidates for dialysis based on notions of social worth, prompted a renewed interest in the ethical basis for medical practice. At the same time there was a shift in the focus of academic moral philosophy from a pre-occupation with metaethical questions (e.g., are moral 'facts' the same kind of thing as scientific 'facts'?, what is the status of moral laws?, etc.) to an interest in normative ethics (e.g. is there such a thing as a 'just war'?, is vegetarianism morally preferable?, etc.). This shift was caused by several factors, not the least of which was an influx of young philosophers with connections to the student movements of the time; many of these were unemployed and looked for a niche in which philosophy and activism could be gainfully combined. These two separate developments coalesced to form the field we now recognise as bioethics [1–3].

Measured in volume, bioethics is a tremendous success. Every year new journals are created and are able to attract articles, new bioethics programmes are started at universities, and many more people get postgraduate degrees in the field. However, in recent years both internal and external criticism has been raised about the subjects being pursued, the methods used, and the results obtained in bioethics. Specific authors [4], or whole schools of bioethics have been targeted [5].

Fulford et al. remind us that bioethics was originally conceived as an interdisciplinary enterprise, with room for a fruitful interaction between philosophers and practitioners [6]. They lament the move towards what they identify as the 'committee mentality', and write the following about their own experiences:

> Yet our experience in these working parties was largely disappointing. On the safe ground of review there was secure scholarship and sound opinion. But when it came to new ideas, to pushing the subject forward, in place of the anticipated fusion of the disciplines there was often mutual incomprehension. To the doctors, conscious of practical imperatives, the philosophers appeared excessively preoccupied with theory. Philosophical debate with its tendency to diversity of opinion and approach seemed hopelessly inconclusive. To the philosophers, on the other hand, the hopes of the doctors for definite answers, for solutions to the particular difficulties posed by the individual concrete cases, seemed unrealistic. Both sides, none the less, were conscious of a pressure to perform: reports had (somehow) to be produced, conclusions (of some kind) had to be published. But the result was an anodyne, an all too familiar compromise of a broadly consequentialist kind, unimpeachable yet often unsatisfying. It was neither sufficiently cognisant of the gritty details faced by professionals at the clinical coal-face, nor adequately addressed to the full interest and subtlety

of the theoretical issues embodied by these same dilemmas [6, pp. 1–2].

This quote draws together two common themes in many of the complaints about the development of bioethics: bioethical theory is too simple-minded, and bioethicists do not take sufficient account of the realities of clinical practice. I tend to agree with both complaints, but would add as a third that a great part of bioethics scholarship exhibits a curious neglect towards the fact that the actions prescribed by bioethicists must be carried out by actual human beings with an independent mind and independent moral reasoning; and that these human beings (also known as health care professionals) work within elaborate organisational structures which constrain their actions in various ways.

This work is an attempt to address a small part of this neglect through an empirical study of the moral reasoning of health care personnel and the influence of hierarchical structures in medicine on treatment decisions with an ethical component.

Outline of the book

Thematically, the empirical study described in the second part of this book belongs to a category of studies usually labelled empirical ethics. Within moral philosophy there is great controversy about the value of such studies and the use of their results. Are they merely an advanced form of opinion poll telling us what people presently think and feel, or are they useful to our deliberations about how people *ought to* think and feel? [7] This topic will be discussed in Chapter 2.

The empirical study is based on what is usually called qualitative research methods – that is, methods based on elucidation of the meaning of human expressions or acts. The scientific status of such methods is grudgingly accepted in sociology, psychology, and often enthusiastically enunciated by nursing scientists, but within medical science it is still very much in dispute. In Chapter 3 I will try to make a small contribution to this debate, by pointing to ways in which arguments from the philosophy of science can bring some clarification to the status and promise of qualitative methods.

After these initial clarifications, Chapter 4 explains why the empirical research was designed and performed as it was, and reports part of the results. Chapter 5 reports another part of the results and integrates them into a discussion of the influence of health care organisation on ethical decision-making. A tentative synthesis of the results is attempted in Chapter 6, but, to the persistent reader who reaches that far, it will be evident, that this is a field where there is still a lot of work to be done.

Because the empirical study reported here involves sociological and ethnographical data-collection methods, qualitative data analysis methods, and subject-matter from moral philosophy, moral psychology, sociology of medicine, and organisational studies, it has been necessary to leave out a lot of interesting theoretical and methodological issues ranging from questions about the relevance of moral philosophy in a postmodern world on the one hand to questions about the scientific validity of non-standardised, not fully structured interviews on the other. This is neither because I believe that these problems are of any less intrinsic interest, nor because I believe they have been satisfactorily solved, but primarily because a thorough treatment of all the interesting questions raised would require many more pages than are available here.

Moral reasoning and moral action

This is a study of the moral attitudes and the moral reasoning of health care professionals (nurses and doctors). It tries to describe and explain how these persons identify ethical problems, how they reason about them, and how the organisational structures of the health care system influences these processes. It is not a direct study of the actual actions that health care personnel perform in response to ethically problematic situations. Such a study of moral action would be immensely valuable, but raises ethical problems about the consent of the patients, and practical problems in getting the relevant access and cooperation.

James Rest has pointed out that there are at least four steps in the process from the identification of an ethical problem to an appropriate ethical action, and that a focus on moral reasoning only covers one of these steps [8, 9]:

> 1. The person must have been able to make some sort of interpretation of the particular situation in terms of what actions were possible, who (including oneself) would be affected by each course of action, and how the interested parties would regard such effects on their welfare.
>
> 2. The person must have been able to make a judgement about which course of action was morally right (or fair or just or morally good), thus labeling one possible line of action as what a person ought (morally ought) to do in that situation.
>
> 3. The person must give priority to moral values above other personal values such that a decision is made to intend to do what is morally right.
>
> 4. The person must have sufficient perseverance, ego strength, and implementation skills to be able to follow through on his/her intention to behave morally, to withstand fatigue and flagging will, and to overcome obstacles [9, pp. 3–4].

Blum identifies 7 steps in this process [10], partly overlapping the steps identified by Rest:

> 1. Accurate recognition of a situation's features.
> 2. Recognising the features that are morally significant.
> 3. Moving from moral characterisation of the situation to the question of whether one should take action.
> 4. Judging whether one should in fact take action.
> 5. Selection of the rule or principle which is applicable to the situation.
> 6. Determining the act that best instantiates the rule or principle.
> 7. Deciding how to perform the act.

Blum repeatedly stresses that correct identification of a moral problem and correct moral reasoning do not guarantee correct moral action. There may be intervening non-moral factors that prevent an agent from doing what he or she knows to be morally right; there may be moral factors that did not reach the level of consciousness when the problem was first consid-ered [11]; or the agent may just choose not to do that action that he or she knows is good and right. The complex of ques-tions concerning the connection between moral reasoning and moral action has traditionally been discussed in ethical theory under the rubric of 'akratic failure' or 'weakness of will' (that is, why do people not do right even when they know it to be right). It is well known that Socrates held the radical doctrine that anyone who knows what is right will also do what is right, but this point of view has never been widely accepted. The intricacies and historical development of this debate are not important here (for a well-informed discussion of this problem see Robert Audi's *Practical Reasoning*) [12]; what is important is the question that the debate raises, namely, why should we study the identification of ethical problems and moral reason-ing if there is no direct link between correct identification and reasoning and correct action?

The first important point to remember is that although correct moral reasoning does not automatically lead to correct moral action, there is nevertheless some connection between the two. If we imagine a situation in which an agent is con-fronted with a moral problem, it will usually be the case that he or she is more likely to choose the right action if this action is also the one that her or his deliberations point to as the morally right action. Most agents have a basic desire to do that which is morally right. The origin of this desire may be sus-pect if one adheres to psychoanalytic theory, but it is, none the less, a desire that most agents express and act upon. We would think that a person was either seriously mentally deranged, or evil in the true sense of this word, if he or she consistently chose to perform those acts which he or she knew to be morally wrong.

The second point, which is especially important in the health care field, is that in the education, and concomitant socialisation of health care workers a professional obligation to 'do that which is right' is reinforced. In the professional set-ting 'that which is right' is not always co-extensional with 'that which is morally right', but it usually includes injunctions against doing 'that which is morally wrong'. This professional obligation may therefore further reinforce the connection between moral reasoning and moral action.

Conversely, it is difficult to see how an agent could consistently perform morally right actions without some form of moral reasoning. We can perhaps imagine somebody who is instinctually virtuous, and who always chooses the right action without any prior thought, but this picture does not seem to be valid for most human beings. Most of us, at least occasionally, have to engage in moral reasoning to be able to choose the morally right action.

In institutional settings, and in the formulation of public, policy moral reasoning attains independent importance. We require our leaders to be able to provide a rationale for the policies they promote, and we are usually not satisfied with the answer 'because it is the right thing to do'. Those in a position to influence institutional or public policy in ethically contentious areas will therefore need to be able to engage in moral reasoning (or at least to give the impression that they are).

These considerations point to a moderate conclusion. Even if we knew all there was to know about the identification of ethical problems and about moral reasoning, we would not be able to predict a person's action accurately. But, compared to a situation in which we knew nothing about these subjects our predictive powers would probably be increased.

The present state of knowledge

A basic premise of the present study is that our knowledge of how health care professionals (and other human beings) reason about ethical issues is not sufficient, and that current conceptualisations in moral psychology are problematic. If this was not the case, the study would be rather uninteresting.

This may come as a surprise to some. In the literature it is easy to find psychometric scales measuring 'moral development', 'moral orientation', or 'moral attitudes' (for a relatively recent review see [13]). It would be reasonable to suppose that before setting out to measure something, you would have a reasonable idea about the content and limits of the thing you are going to measure, but this is not really the case in moral psychology. Here, two other approaches seem to be more common. Either you have an ethical theory and you develop an instrument which measures conformance to the theory, or you have empirical data describing a developmental sequence in moral reasoning, and you develop an instrument based on these data with later developmental stages representing better moral reasoning.

An extreme example of the first approach is the Hartman Value Profile, which is based on a complete value algebra developed by R. S. Hartman [14–16]. This instrument undoubtedly measures whether the moral reasoning of the respondents follows the rules prescribed by Hartmanian value algebra, but given that the theoretical assumptions underlying this approach to ethics are rejected by most moral philosophers (and I suspect by most other people as well), the knowledge that is gained is of no great value. Similar attempts, taking their theoretical framework from more generally accepted theories of ethics, would be more valuable, but would still only measure conformance with one or, at best, a limited number of ethical theories, and there seems to be no a priori reason to assume that actual moral reasoning is congruent with ethical theory.

The second approach is probably best exemplified by Kohlberg's cognitive-developmental theory and Gilligan's alternative care ethic approach (see below). The Kohlberg–Gilligan controversy has played a major role in the discussions of moral reasoning, moral psychology, and moral development in the last ten to fifteen years, and has had a great impact on the development of feminist and nursing ethics.

I have, however, decided to use neither of these two approaches in the analysis of the present data. In the following sections I shall try to explain the reasoning behind this rejection. They do not constitute a full review of the extensive literature about these theories (the recent *Handbook of Moral Behavior and Development*, which is itself mainly a review, contains three volumes and about 1,200 pages of text) [17], but they are targeted specifically at the use of these theories and the instruments developed to measure their central constructs in non-interventional studies involving adult health care personnel.

Apart from Kohlberg's and Gilligan's works the social learning theory of moral development championed by Bandura and Walters [18] and, more recently, social cognitive theory [19] have also been influential. Social cognitive theory has never really been used in the health care field, maybe because its research paradigm focuses primarily on experimental studies, where variables, such as degree of external pressure, can be manipulated and the effect of the manipulation measured in terms of different actions. Such experimental studies could conceivably be performed in the health care setting, but it would probably be considerably more difficult to recruit and deceive health care personnel than to recruit and deceive the high school and college students who are the usual objects of the psychologists' experiments.

Kohlberg and cognitive-developmental theory

Lawrence Kohlberg (1927–87) is undoubtedly the most important figure in modern moral psychology, and much of the academic discussion is still put in terms of being for or against him. The main claims in the classic formulation of his theory are (see the essays collected in [20]):

1. moral development involves change in cognitive structures, similar to the changes involved in acquiring logical concepts;
2. moral development progresses through a single unitary set of stages, although development may be arrested at any of these;
3. the path of moral development is the same in different cultures and for the two genders.

Kohlberg developed his theory in the 1950s, based on a longitudinal study of a sample of boys [21], from which he identified three levels of morality – preconventional, conventional, postconventional – each consisting of two stages [modified from 20, vol. 1, p. 128]:

Stage 1:   Obedience and punishment orientation
Stage 2:   Instrumental hedonism and exchange
Stage 3:   Orientation to approval and stereotypes of virtue
Stage 4:   Law and order orientation
Stages 5–6:   Orientation to principles of justice and welfare

Progression between the stages is seen as involving the acquisition, understanding, and use of a more and more abstract conception of justice. In one of his papers Kohlberg presents the following table, where the stages are exemplified by the conception of the moral worth of human life held by persons at a given stage [modified from 20, vol. 1, pp. 118–20]:

Stage 1:   There is no differentiation between the moral value of life and its physical or social status value.

Stage 2:   Value of a human life is seen as instrumental to satisfaction of the needs of its possessor or others. Decision to save life is relative to, or to be made by, its possessor. (There is differentiation of physical and interest value of life, of its value to self and to others.)

Stage 3:   Value of a human life is based on empathy and affection of family and others toward its possessor. (Value is based on social sharing, community, love; differentiated from instrumental and hedonistic value applicable also to animals.)

Stage 4:   Life is conceived as sacred in terms of its place in a categorial moral or religious order of rights and duties. (Value is in relation to a moral order, differentiated from value to specific others in family, and so on. Value still partly depends, however, on serving the group, the state, God, and so on.)

Stage 5:   Life valued both in terms of its relation to community welfare and in terms of being a universal human right. (Obligation to respect the basic right to life is differentiated from generalised respect for the sociomoral order. General value of the independent human life is a primary autonomous value, not dependent on other values.)

Stage 6:   Human life is sacred because of the universal prin-
           ciple of respect for the individual. (Moral value of a
           human being, as an object of moral principle, is dif-
           ferentiated from a formal recognition of his or her
           rights.)

Kohlberg also developed an instrument for measuring moral
development, based on responses prompted by hypothetical
stories involving moral dilemmas. The Kohlberg instrument
requires a face-to-face interview, with a full transcription, and
scoring by a trained scorer (the present scoring manual is over
500 pages long) [22]. Because of these practical constraints the
instrument has not been very much used by researchers outside the Kohlberg group.

Subsequently, Rest developed a paper-and-pen instrument
– Defining Issues Test (DIT)) – building on the same paradigm [8, 9]. DIT can be scored automatically by a computer,
and has therefore become the instrument of choice for measuring moral development within this tradition. A recent
volume of reviews on the use of DIT reports numerous studies concerning high school, college, and university students,
schoolteachers, doctors, nurses, dentists, veterinarians, accoun-
tants, journalists, and athletes, all of whom can be shown to
develop higher DIT scores in circumstances where moral
development is to be expected [23]. DIT has also influenced
nursing research through the development of Crisham's Nursing Dilemmas Test, which runs parallel to DIT, using dilemmas from nursing practice [24].

All three instruments mentioned above are well validated,
and probably do measure the central construct of cognitive-
developmental theory fairly accurately – that is, they measure
the degree to which respondents use an abstract conception of
justice in their moral deliberations. There are minor technical
problems with the Kohlberg and Rest instruments, because
some of the dilemma stories used have become slightly dated
(e.g. DIT uses a story about the Vietnam war and reserve officer training), but these are not sufficient to invalidate the
instruments. There are, however, two theoretical questions

which need to be addressed: first, do the instruments measure the right thing – that is, is development of the central construct in cognitive-developmental theory really congruent with moral development? Second, do the instruments map the whole of the moral domain?

The first question has been extensively addressed in the literature. Kohlberg himself linked his theory to the moral theories of Kant (that is, the American version of Kant without the transcendental element), Rawls, and Hare, and claimed that there were good philosophical arguments showing that higher stages exemplify a more adequate mode of moral reasoning than lower stages. It is obvious that the highly abstract conception of justice used in the higher stages have affinities to the formal nature of Kant's moral philosophy and to Rawlsian deliberation behind a veil of ignorance, whereas the view of morality as prescriptive and universal, which is also part of stage 6, shows strong similarities to Hare's universal prescriptivism [25–7].

It should not come as a surprise that Kohlberg's ideas about justice shows congruence with philosophical ideas about justice. Aristotle defined justice in a formal sense as 'treating equal cases equally', and there has not been much improvement on this formula since then. The real discussion is, however, about substantive justice. What factors make cases equal, and what is equal treatment?

Kohlberg's conception of justice and moral development give few answers to these questions. The formal agreement between his conception of justice and some leading moral theories is not followed by a substantive agreement about what kind of things or goods this conception should be applied to. This is not surprising. There is, for instance, a great difference between Rawls and Hare in the kind of goods they see as important. Hare argues that morality is really about the maximisation of preference satisfaction, whereas Rawls specifies a list of primary goods that must be distributed according to rules of justice. There is no way to unite these two different theories on the substantive level. This means that the formal similarities in the conception of justice may be accompanied by totally different decisions in concrete moral problems. Within Kohlberg's framework, there is no way to adjudicate these differences if we assume that they both follow from the perfect, stage 6 mode of reasoning. It follows that we may accept that development according to Kohlberg's instrument is true moral development, and still claim that stage 6 people are not fully morally developed. They may have the right mode of reasoning, but the wrong content in their theory of values or in their metaethics.

This is where the second problem becomes important, when one accepts that the development in the justice perspective that Kohlberg describes is really a positive development, but asks the question: 'Is this really all there is, or is there more to morality than formal justice?' Some traditional virtues, like courage, compassion, or benevolence, do not seem to find any room in this conception of morality, and there is no place in the higher stages (above stage 3) for recognition of the moral importance of special relationships (e.g., parent–child, doctor–patient, etc.).

The description of the higher stages, and especially stage 6, shows a prime example of a morality advocating the detached view from nowhere as the only proper view to take. Kohlberg's conception of morality is therefore open to all the objections raised against agent-neutral moralities advanced by Nagel and Scheffler [28, 29] — that is, that agent-neutral moralities fail to take account of important moral facts created by human relationships, and that they prescribe a morality so stringent, and a motivational structure so alien, that the result is a morality unfit for humans. These objections are usually raised against versions of act-consequentialism. Kohlberg strongly denies that his position is directly consequentialist, but the core of the objections is valid against any moral theory not admitting the relevance of agent-specific considerations, whether or not the theory is consequentialist. This has led Barry to argue that the core errors in Kohlberg's theory are a failure to distinguish between first and second order impartiality, and the elevation of first order impartiality to the level of an absolute principle [30].

Within the cognitive-developmental paradigm any statement of an agent-specific moral consideration or any statement
propounding classical virtues, are scored as evidence of a lower
level of moral development, and will therefore subtract from
the respondents' moral stage. Or, to put it differently, all considerations not conforming to the abstract justice perspective of
stages 5–6 are scored as lack of development or errors.

The instruments developed in the cognitive-developmental
theory tradition are therefore not of much use in explorative
studies of how people actually think about morality. They do
measure how the respondents use the concept of justice, but
they do not tell anything about other aspects of the respondents' moral reasoning, because these aspects are either
ignored or subsumed in the final score as 'error'.

One could, of course, perform interviews using the
Kohlberg moral judgement interview guide and then analyse
them without applying cognitive-developmental theory, but
the advantage of such a strategy is difficult to see.

The 'Ethic of Care' approach

'Ethic of care' is the name of a rapidly expanding school of
thought which began as a phenomenon in nursing ethics and
feminist ethics, but has now spread to all areas of health care
ethics. The beginning of a modern ethics of care can be traced
to the publication of Carol Gilligan's book *In a Different Voice*
in 1982 [31]. In this book she criticises classical moral psychology and cognitive-developmental theory as it had been
developed by her mentor Lawrence Kohlberg (see above), and
claims that her research shows that men and women follow
different developmental paths. The last claim has since been
modified and weakened to state that men and women on average use different moral orientations [32].

In two articles in the second edition of the *Encyclopedia of
Bioethics*, Reich traces the historical roots of the concept of care
and its use in ethics, and shows how it was used before 1982
[33, 34]. Despite his convincing argument that its use in ethics
can be traced back to the Stoics, there is no doubt that the
modern ethic of care movement is largely unaware of and

unconcerned with these earlier developments. When non-contemporary philosophers are cited in the ethic of care literature it is almost always as examples of opposing and restricted views which an ethic of care has now overcome. There are of course exceptions to this rule [35], but these are few and far between. For practical purposes it is therefore legitimate to trace the modern ethic of care back no further than to Gilligan's 1982 book.

Gilligan presents two main criticisms of Kohlberg. The first is methodological and is directed towards the fact that his theory has been developed from a longitudinal study of a sample consisting only of boys. The second is substantive and claims that, partly as a result of the decision to omit girls from the sample, the theory overlooks an important area of the moral domain, namely the moral experiences of women. Kohlberg's theory sees moral development as a step towards the use of a progressively more abstract theory of justice; Gilligan's argument is that this is only part of the moral realm. Based on her own studies of girls and young women, she claims that their development can be understood much better if seen not in terms of an abstract theory of justice, but in terms of relationship or care. Gilligan retains the developmental scheme with three developmental levels, but she gives them an entirely new content. Her book sparked off an ongoing debate in moral psychology, feminist theory, and moral philosophy, and has been very influential in the development of the ethic of care.

Later empirical research using Gilligan's framework has further complicated matters. It is now clear that justice and care are not mutually exclusive in the sense that a given person only uses one of these approaches. Most people shift freely between the two positions, and whereas it is true that women use the care orientation more than men, men are usually fully proficient in its use [36–38]. Furthermore, it has been shown, that the type of moral dilemma used to elicit the response to a large extent determines which orientation is chosen. Personal dilemmas predispose people to use the care orientation, whereas impersonal dilemmas more often elicit a justice response [39–41]. Women are more prone to relate personal experiences when asked to describe a moral dilemma they have experienced, and some researchers have suggested that this alone may explain the gender differences found in moral orientation [41].

Theoretically, the concept of care has been developed beyond the initial ideas put forward by Gilligan, and today it is probably a mistake to talk about *the* concept of care, since different scholars have developed very different conceptualisations. A 1991 review article of theories of caring in nursing science lists twenty-three different conceptualisations of care and caring found in Anglo-American nursing literature, and groups them in five distinct categories [42]:

1. caring as a human trait;
2. caring as a moral imperative;
3. caring as an affect;
4. caring as an interpersonal interaction;
5. caring as therapeutic intervention.

Outside the health care field, in general moral philosophy and in feminist ethics, an even more confusing array of options can be found, and although many are happy to talk about an ethic of care, it is fairly evident that there is no real agreement on what care actually is. Authors easily identify specific instances of care, and specific situations requiring a caring response, but the move from such instances to a more theoretical notion creates an almost bewildering range of different proposals [43, 44].

Within the field, one can find discussions about whether justice and care are really distinct or whether one of the approaches can subsume the other [45, 47]; discussions about whether an ethic of care is necessarily a women's ethics [48, 49]; discussions about whether justice and care are simply labels for the morality of two distinct spheres of human interaction, the justice orientation being appropriate for the public sphere where we interact with strangers, and the care orientation being appropriate for the private sphere where we interact with intimates [50, 51]; discussions about whether 'ethic of care' is in itself just a preliminary and discardable label for a larger field of non-principle-based particularist ethics, or a label for a subsection of this field alongside virtue ethics, narrative ethics, etc. [52]; and discussions about whether the character traits in the ethic of care that we normally consider to be good and admirable really ought to be so valorised. If these character traits had developed historically as adaptations or survival strategies by the oppressed (that is, women) in patriarchal society, they may not be valuable at all *sub specie aeternitatis* [53].

There are no signs that these debates are getting nearer to closure, and recent work in the field has been far more successful in flagging the problems and questions than in providing convincing answers [54, 55]. Several problems therefore arise when one tries to use the ethic of care approach as an analytic guide in an empirical study of moral reasoning. First, one has to choose one specific conception of care among the many available. Second, one has to construct an instrument for measuring or assessing this conception so as to make it useful in empirical research. Apart from Gilligan's work, and empirical work by other researchers directly related to it [36, 37], there are no such instruments to be found in the literature.

This state of affairs seems to be caused by two almost contradictory factors. On the one hand, some empirical researchers seem to believe that the content of the concept of care is easily definable or self-evident and that it is therefore not necessary to construct any specific instrument for assessing this concept. On the other, many of the conceptions of care put forward in the theoretical literature are so vague or have such fuzzy borders that it is either impossible to make any instrument for their assessment, or impossible to do so in a way that distinguishes care from closely related notions like professional responsibility.

This two-sided problem leads to an unfortunate situation in which empirical researchers interested in moral reasoning are left with three not very appealing options: a) to accept Gilligan's concept of care and work with the available instrument for assessing this specific conception; b) to develop a useful instrument of measuring or assessing one of the other available conceptions of care; c) to develop a whole new concept of care, including a new instrument for assesing it, from the data collected.

The first option is unappealing because there are good methodological and philosophical arguments against accepting Gilligan's specific concept of care [56]. On further analysis it turns out to be less clearly defined than could be wished, and less clearly distinguishable from justice considerations [10].

The second may well turn out to be a Sisyphean task, and the third option is not appealing to the researcher who wants to get a tool or who believes that care is only one (perhaps small) part of the ethical landscape.

In a study of the moral reasoning and attitudes of health care personnel further problems occur because a number of nursing theorists have developed arguments which claim that caring, as defined by the theory, is unique to nursing [42]. If one accepts this somewhat surprising claim, an instrument for assessing such a concept of care would only be applicable to studies of nurses and not to those involving other health care professionals, unless of course the purpose of the study was to disprove or support the theoretical contention of uniqueness. I must admit that I find it difficult to see how the concept of caring could be unique to nursing, unless it was totally dislodged from our common understanding of caring, and I fully agree with Benner and Wrubel in their statement that: 'Caring practices are lived out in this culture primarily in parenting, child care, nursing, education, counseling and various forms of community life' [57, p. 408].

During the initial analysis of the interviews in the present study the concept of care and its development within a number of theories of an ethic of care was kept in mind, but, given the reliance on grounded theory methodology, it was not forced upon the data. The initial analysis yielded no categories which can be mapped directly on to the concept of care, but the core category which did emerge – 'protective responsibility' – obviously has some connections with different aspects of the concept of care. These connections and their theoretical ramifications are briefly explored in Chapter 4.

References

1 Toulmin, S., How medicine saved the life of ethics. *Perspectives in Biology and Medicine* 1978; 25(4): 736–50.

2 Fox, R. C., The evolution of American bioethics: a sociological perspective. In: George Weisz (ed.), *Social Science Perspectives on Medical Ethics*. Philadelphia: University of Pensylvania Press, 1990: pp. 202–17.

3 Rothman, D. J., *Strangers at the Bedside: A History of how Law and Bioethics Transformed Medical Decision Making*. New York: Basic Books, 1991.

4 Maclean, A., *The Elimination of Morality: Reflections on Utilitarianism and Bioethics*. London: Routledge, 1993.

5 Holm, S., American bioethics at the crossroads – a critical appraisal. *European Philosophy of Medicine and Health Care* 1994; 2(2): 6–23.

6 Fulford, K. W. M., Gillett, G., Soskice, J. M., Introduction: diverse ethics. In: Fulford, Gillett, and Soskice (eds), *Medicine and Moral Reasoning*. Cambridge: Cambridge University Press, 1994: pp. 1–5.

7 Flanagan, O., Rorty, A. O., Introduction. In: Flanagan and Rorty (eds), *Identity, Character, and Morality: Essays in Moral Psychology*. Cambridge, MA: MIT Press, 1990: pp. 1–15.

8 Rest, J., *Development in Judging Moral Issues*. Minneapolis: University of Minnesota Press, 1979.

9 Rest, J., Bebeau, M., Volker, J., An overview of the psychology of morality. In: Rest, J. (ed.), *Moral Development: Advances in Research and Theory*. New York: Praeger, 1986: pp. 1–27.

10 Blum, L. A., *Moral Perception and Particularity*. New York: Cambridge University Press, 1994: pp. 58–61.

11 McIntyre, A., Is akratic action always irrational? In: Flanagan, O., Rorty, A. O. (eds), *Identity, Character, and Morality: Essays in Moral Psychology*. Cambridge, MA: MIT Press, 1990: pp. 379–400.

12 Audi, R., *Practical Reasoning*. London: Routledge, 1989.

13 Waterman A. S., On the uses of psychological theory and research in the process of ethical inquiry. *Psychological Bulletin* 1988; 103(3): 283–98.

14 Hartman, R. S., *The Structure of Value: Foundations of Scientific Axiology*. Carbondale, IL: Southern Illinois University Press, 1967.

15 Hartman, R. S., *The Hartman Value Profile (HVP) Manual of Interpretation*. Muskegon, MI: Research Concepts, 1973.

16 Forrest, F. G., *Valuemetrics: The Science of Personal and Professional*

Ethics, Value Inquiry Book Series (vol. 11). Amsterdam: Rodopi, 1994.

17 Kurtines, W. M., Gewirtz, J. L. (eds), H*andbook of Moral Behavior and Development* (3 vols). Hillsdale, NJ: Lawrence Erlbaum Associates, 1991.

18 Bandura, A., Walters, R. H., *Adolescent Aggression*. New York; Ronald Press, 1959.

19 Bandura, A., *Social Foundations of Thought and Action: A Social Cognitive Theory*. Englewood Cliffs, NJ: Prentice-Hall, 1986.

20 Kohlberg, L., *Essays in Moral Development* (2 vols). New York: Harper and Row, 1982/84.

21 Kohlberg, L., The development of modes of thinking and choices in years 10 to 16. Unpublished Ph.D. dissertation, University of Chicago, 1958.

22 Colby, A., Kohlberg, L., *The Measurement of Moral Judgement* (2 vols). Cambridge: Cambridge University Press, 1987.

23 Rest, J. R., Narváez, D. (eds), *Moral Development in the Professions – Psychology and Applied Ethics*. Hillsdale, NJ: Lawrence Erlbaum Associates, 1994.

24 Crisham, P., Measuring moral judgment in nursing dilemmas. *Nursing Research* 1982; 30(2): 104–10.

25 Kant, I., *Grundlegung zur Methaphysik der Sitten*. Hamburg: Felix Meiner Verlag, 1965 (first published 1785).

26 Rawls, J., A *Theory of Justice*. Oxford: Oxford University Press, 1972.

27 Hare, R. M., *The Language of Morals*. Oxford: Clarendon Press, 1952.

28 Nagel, T., *The View from Nowhere*. New York: Oxford University Press, 1986.

29 Scheffler, S., *Human Morality*. New York: Oxford University Press, 1992.

30 Barry, B., *Justice as Impartiality*. Oxford: Clarendon Press, 1995.

31 Gilligan, C., In *a Different Voice: Psychological Theory and Women's Development.* Cambridge, MA: Harvard University Press, 1982.

32 Gilligan, C., Moral orientation and moral development. In: Kittay, E. F., Meyers, D. T. (eds), *Women and Moral Theory*. New York: Rowman and Littlefield, 1987: pp. 19–33.

33 Reich, W. T., Care: I. History of the notion of care. In: Reich (ed.), *Encyclopedia of Bioethics* (2nd edn). New York: Simon and Schuster Macmillan, 1995: pp. 319–31.

34 Reich, W. T., Care: II. Historical dimensions of an ethic of care in health care. In: Reich (ed.), *Encyclopedia of Bioethics* (2nd edn). New York: Simon and Schuster Macmillan, 1995: pp. 331–6.

35 Baier, A. C., Hume, the women's moral theorist. In: Kittay, E. F., Meyers, D. T. (eds), *Women and Moral Theory*. New York: Rowman and Littlefield, 1987: pp. 37–55.

36 Lyons, N. P., Two perspectives: on self, relationships, and morality. *Harvard Educational Review* 1983; 53(2): 125–45.

37 Gilligan, C., Attanucci, C., Two moral orientations: gender differences and similarities. *Merrill-Palmer Quarterly* 1988; 34(3): 223–37.

38 Stiller, N. J., Forrest, L., An extension of Gilligan and Lyon's investigation of morality: gender differences in college students. *Journal of College Student Development* 1990; 31: 54–63.

39 Pratt, M. W., Golding, G., Hunter, W., Sampson, R., Sex differences in adult moral orientations. *Journal of Personality* 1988; 56(2): 373–91.

40 Walker, L. J., de Vries, B., Trevethan, S. D., Moral stages and moral orientation in real-life and hypothetical dilemmas. *Child Development* 1987; 58: 842–858.

41 Walker, L. J., A longitudinal study of moral reasoning. *Child Development* 1989; 60: 157–66.

42 Morse, J. M., Bottorf, J., Neander, W., Solberg, S., Comparative analysis of conceptualizations and theories of caring. *IMAGE: Journal of Nursing Scholarship* 1991; 23(2): 119–26.

43 Ruddick, S., *Maternal Thinking: Toward a Politics of Peace*. New York: Ballantine Books, 1989.

44 Noddings, N., *Caring*. Berkeley: University of California Press, 1984.

45 Baier, A. C., The need for more than justice. *Canadian Journal of Philosophy* 1987; 13(suppl.): 41–56.

46 Stocker, M., Duty and friendship: toward a synthesis of Gilligan's contrastive moral concepts. In: Kittay, E. F., Meyers, D. T. (eds), *Women and Moral Theory*. New York: Rowman and Littlefield, 1987: pp. 56–68.

47 Sher, G., Other voices, other rooms? Women's psychology and moral theory. In: Kittay, E. F., Meyers, D. T. (eds), *Women and Moral Theory*. New York: Rowman and Littlefield, 1987: pp. 178–89.

48 Held, V., Feminism and moral theory. In: Kittay, E. F., Meyers, D. T. (eds), *Women and Moral Theory*. New York: Rowman and Littlefield, 1987: pp. 111–28)

49 Fox, E. L., Seeing through women's eyes: the role of vision in women's moral theory. In: Cole, E. B., Coultrap-McQuin, S. (eds), *Explorations in Feminist Ethics: Theory and Practice*. Bloomington: Indiana University Press, 1992: pp. 111–6.

50 Sommers, C. H., Filial morality. *The Journal of Philosophy* 1986; 83(8): 439–56.

51 Dillon, R. S., Care and Respect. In: Cole, E. B., Coultrap-McQuin, S. (eds), *Explorations in Feminist Ethics: Theory and Practice*. Bloomington: Indiana University Press, 1992: pp. 69–81.

52 Sharpe, V. A., Justice and care: the implications of the Kohlberg–Gilligan

debate for medical ethics. *Theoretical Medicine* 1992; 13: 295–318.

53 Card, C., Gender and moral luck. In: Flanagan, O., Rorty, A. O. (eds), *Identity, Character, and Morality: Essays in Moral Psychology*. Cambridge, MA: MIT Press, 1990: pp. 199–218.

54 Romain, D., Care and confusion. In: Cole, E. B., Coultrap-McQuin, S. (eds), *Explorations in Feminist Ethics: Theory and Practice*. Bloomington: Indiana University Press, 1992: pp. 27–37.

55 Tronto, J. C., *Moral Boundaries: A Political Argument for an Ethic of Care*. New York: Routledge, 1993.

56 Smith, J. A., Abortion and moral development theory: listening with different ears. *International Philosophical Quarterly* 1988; 28(1): 31–51.

57 Benner, P., Wrubel, J., *The Primacy of Caring: Stress and Coping in Health and Illness*. Menlo Park, CA: Addison Wesley, 1989.

2

Engaging the world: a defence of descriptive ethics

If medical ethics is to take and hold a central place in the practice of medicine, it is vital that it should build up a body of empirical data to reduce its reliance on conjecture. Yet it remains rare to find contributions to such data in bioethics journals. Instead they are scattered through the general medical journals [1, p. 16].

Introduction

In recent years we have seen a rapid increase in the number of articles reporting empirical studies of ethical attitudes, ethical reasoning, ethical actions, or the understanding of the words used in ethical arguments. This trend can be observed in both bioethics and in business ethics, but the present chapter will primarily be concerned with the former, although arguments from the business ethics literature on the proper relationship between normative and descriptive ethics will also be considered. A large problem, which will not be considered here, is the scientific quality of the extant empirical ethical studies, and the proper research methodology to apply (that is, quantitative versus qualitative studies). A 'medical' answer to these questions can be found in [2], and a more balanced view in [3].

Traditionally, studies of ethical attitudes have been called descriptive ethics, and have been placed on the lowest rung of the three-part division consisting of descriptive ethics, normative ethics, and metaethics. In the philosophical literature the role of descriptive ethics is often downplayed. In the fourth edition of the influential *The Principles of Biomedical Ethics* by Beauchamp and Childress we read: 'Often in this book we cite descriptive ethics – for example, by presenting what professional codes require. However, the underlying question is usually whether the described prescriptions of such codes are defensible, which is a normative issue' [4, p. 5]. And this is just a moderate restatement of Sidgwick's claim that:

> On any theory, our view of what ought to be must be largely derived, in details, from our apprehension of what is; the means of realising our ideal can only be thoroughly learnt by a careful study of actual phenomena; and to any individual asking himself 'What ought I to do or aim at?' it is important to examine the answers which his fellow-men have actually given to similar questions. Still it seems clear that an attempt to ascertain the general laws or uniformities by which the varieties of human conduct, and of men's sentiments and judgments respecting conduct, may be *explained*, is essentially different from an attempt to determine which among these varieties of conduct is *right* and which of these divergent judgments *valid* [5, p. 2, emphasis in the original].

Moral philosophers have held that to give empirical descriptions normative status would be to derive an 'ought' from an 'is' – that is, to commit the naturalistic fallacy. This diagnosis is probably correct if the empirical statements are of the type '69 per cent of the inhabitants of Mauritania accept slavery', but, as we shall see, it may be wrong for statements such as 'It is psychologically impossible for humans to be totally impartial'.

The sociological reasons for the resurgence of descriptive ethics are fairly straightforward. Bioethics is a multi-disciplinary field, and those bioethicists who come to it from medicine, nursing, psychology, or sociology bring along their own professional traditions, which generally hold empirical research in high esteem.

From a philosophical perspective the resurgence is, at first sight, more puzzling. If it is the case that descriptive ethics is a subject with so little importance that it can be handled in a few sentences in the first chapter of books on ethics, why would anyone then bother to do these studies, which are often elaborate and time-consuming, and explicitly label them 'bioethics' rather than 'sociology of medicine' or 'medical anthropology'? This chapter is an attempt to show that empirical data in general, and descriptive ethics in particular, are potentially much more important in bioethical analysis than is normally acknowledged.

In an article on clinical medical ethics Siegler *et al.* suggest that empirical research in medical ethics can have four purposes: '[it] can help to identify key issues, frame research questions, structure ethical analyses, and contribute to a better understanding of the normative issues that lie at the heart of clinical medical ethics' [6, p. 7]. As will be clear from what follows, I agree with the authors that these four purposes are important, but I argue that we ought to add four more. Two of these are concerned with the pragmatic side of bioethics, because empirical investigations can test the effects of regulations and interventions as well as the effect of teaching bioethics. The other two are on the normative and metaethical level. As I will argue below, empirical studies can bring realism (in the non-metaphysical sense) into ethical analysis, and can investigate which moral theories are compatible with unalterable features of human psychology.

Initial clarifications

The terminology in the field is somewhat confused, and it is necessary to state how I will apply it in this chapter. 'Descriptive ethics' will be used in its classical sense to refer to studies of ethical attitudes; 'moral psychology' will be used to refer to studies of ethical reasoning; 'empirical ethics' will be used for a wider range of studies including those just mentioned as well as studies of the frequency of ethical problems, the effects of regulatory measures, and the effects of teaching ethics; and finally, 'ethics-related studies' will be used for those sociological or psychological studies that aim at clarifying the status of key empirical assumptions in ethical arguments (e.g., do patients really become more anxious when they are fully informed? Would patients really stay away from psychotherapy if they did not believe that confidentiality would be upheld?) [7, 8].

What do you need to do bioethics?

The first thing you need is to know what your purpose is. Are you interested in bioethics because deliberation on the dilemmas in the field may throw new light on interesting theoretical problems in moral philosophy (e.g., ideas about individuation and personhood being sharpened by deliberation on new reproductive techniques), or are you interested in the pragmatic side of bioethics where it impinges more or less directly on health care decisions? This choice will obviously have great importance for the amount of ethics-related studies with which you need to be familiar. The next sections are primarily concerned with the pragmatic side of bioethics, and may therefore be of relatively little interest to those who are only interested in theory. They should, however, be able to find something to suit their taste in the last sections of the chapter.

The second thing you need is a problem, and since bioethics, among other things, distinguishes itself from moral philosophy or ethics in general by having a special subject area, it is from this that the problem must in some way emerge. Problems might come to the attention of the bioethicist in many ways. Legal regulations and court cases have always been a fertile field, as have various exposés of medical scandals. The sole reliance on these sources will, however, give a lopsided view of the ordinary clinical activity of health care professionals.

It may well be that the problems that are philosophically most challenging and interesting are not the ones that are of main interest to health care professionals. They may either be rare, or they may only be present in some small subspecialty of medicine. This creates a problem. If bioethics has nothing to say about the more prevalent and salient ethical problems in medical practice then health care professionals may well lose interest in the pronouncements of the bioethicist. This

alone would indicate that bioethicists have a purely prag-
matic/prudential interest in investigating what kinds of problems health care providers find troublesome.

The importance of knowing something about the frequency, salience, and perceived importance of ethical problems
is further reinforced if we assume that (at least part of) the
purpose of bioethics is to affect changes in the way health care
is delivered, and to minimise the number or gravity of unethical acts towards patients. Simple numerical considerations
seem to indicate that such a purpose is best fulfilled, if the
bioethicist directs her or his efforts towards common ethical
problems.

Realism in bioethics?

The third thing you need to perform a bioethical analysis is
knowledge of the context and environment in which a given
problem occurs. This is not only important in the analysis of
the problem, but also when different 'solutions' are put forward.

Bioethics is sometimes described as 'applied ethics' − you
take your theory and apply it to the case in hand. This model
of bioethics obviously contains many philosophical problems,
as Caplan has shown [9], but it also contains a very practical
problem, because bioethics can never just be applied. It must
also, in a very real sense, be applicable if it is to be of more
than theoretical philosophical interest. Bioethical problems
occur in the real world, they have real world consequences, and
the solutions proposed must be real world solutions. In this
context it is probably wise to remember the words of Dewey:

> Of one thing we may be sure. If inquiries are to have a substantial
> basis, if they are not to be wholly in the air, the theorist must take
> his departure from the problems which men actually meet in their
> own conduct. He may define and refine these; he may divide and
> systematize; he may abstract the problems from their concrete con-
> texts in individual lives; he may classify them when he has thus
> detached them; but if he gets away from them, he is talking about
> something his own brain has invented, not about moral realities
> [10, p. 212].

A lot of the knowledge needed for a realistic analysis of bioethical problems is not gained through empirical ethics or even ethics-related studies; it is simply knowledge about the working conditions in modern health care: how much time is available, who has authority, and what happens to deviants, etc?

We cannot, for instance, expect fully informed consent to be attained in the emergency department, even when the patient is completely conscious, if the working environment does not permit the necessary time to be spent on informing the patient. If time is not available, then the ideal is not attainable, and simply expostulating on the virtues of informed consent will not help anybody. In such a case the focus of the analysis must change from the individual health care provider to the health care delivery system. But this shift is only possible if the bioethicist *knows* that time is not available, and such knowledge can only come from empirical sources, not from philosophical analysis. These sources could consist of medical anecdotes, but as with many other kinds of human activity, medical anecdotes rarely give a true picture of the state of play, and do not amount to a reliable source of information.

A second aspect of the concept of applicability is concerned with the kind of world the philosopher is referring to in her or his analysis. Is it an analysis of the principles applicable in 'the best of all worlds', which in this context must be the world where everybody abides by the moral rules or principles laid down by the philosopher, or, rather, is the analysis intended to say something about how one should act and which principles one should use in a 'less than perfect world' – that is, a world where moral rules and principles vary quite considerably. In utilitarian theory this question is often posed as the question of choosing between conformance and acceptance utility as the measure when laying down moral rules. Where conformance utility is the utility a given rule will generate if all actors act in conformance with the rule, whereas acceptance utility is the utility the rule will generate if all actors accept the rule as a valid moral rule. In the latter case, some actors may not actually act in conformance with the rule, even if they accept it.

There will therefore often be a difference between the conformance and the acceptance utility of a given rule. However, given the moral pluralism of many modern societies we have to go beyond acceptance utility, and talk about pluralistic utility – that is, the utility a given set of rules will have in a world where not everybody accepts them.

In the case of the 'best of all worlds' analysis, no knowledge is needed about present ethical attitudes, because these have no direct relevance for the principles that should be followed in this world. In such a world the moral actions of all actors are predictable because of the uniformity of the moral principles. This means that the consequences[1] of the application of a given principle can be easily calculated.[2]

In an 'almost perfect world', where everyone accepts a single set of moral rules but where these rules are not always obeyed, the case becomes more complicated, but you would still not need descriptive ethics in order to calculate the consequences of a principle. You would only need to know how often and why people acted against the rule.[3]

In a 'less than perfect world' like our own, the same degree of predictability cannot be obtained through purely theoretical considerations. How other people will respond to my actions, and thus the consequences that these actions will have, depends on the moral (and other) attitudes and principles held by other people in my field of action. I can therefore only predict the consequences of following a specific principle, and thereby derivatively only decide what principles to choose/advocate, if I have some knowledge of the attitudes of other people, including knowledge about their moral attitudes. I therefore need descriptive ethics if I want to advocate principles that work in our present world.

Interventions and laws

Bioethicists are often not satisfied with proposing right actions for individual persons. They also propose guidelines, regulations, and laws. But this is again a very problematic enterprise if data from empirical ethical studies are not available. We cannot in general assume that the policies that ought to be promoted should simply directly mimic our notion of right action. If we are interested in abolishing or reducing the number of wrongful actions of a specific kind, it may be necessary and prudent to do more than just prohibit them. Prohibitions have important symbolic functions, but they may not be the most efficient policy instrument.

Baruch Brody has argued that if the moral issue at hand is fundamentally non-consequentialist (e.g., whether we should allow commercialisation of organs) then empirical bioethics research is largely irrelevant and potentially confusing [11]. He argues that in such a case empirical studies can only investigate consequences that are coincidental with the real non-consequentialist core problem. In one sense this is obviously true. We can investigate the harms caused by lying, but not whether lying degrades human dignity. In another sense Brody's claim is not so convincing, because even a non-consequentialist bioethicist could benefit greatly from knowing what factors *caused* physicians to lie to patients, since these causal factors could be a lot more amenable to modification than the physicians' minds. Physicians may be fully aware that what they are doing is morally wrong, but there could be structural or economic factors which prompt them to choose the wrongful action. It is, for instance, very likely that the introduction of a no-fault system for compensation for medical malpractice and mishaps would do more to promote truthfulness in the doctor–patient relationship than any amount of ethical teaching or legal pronouncement.

Many policy analyses proceed from assumptions about what ordinary people want, assumptions about the effect of different kinds of intervention, or assumptions about the motivation of different actors. Unfortunately, such assumptions may be wrong, and the whole analysis thereby misleading. It is not sufficient to assume what the 'person on the Clapham omnibus' thinks, believes, or wants, at least not if it is a matter that could be investigated.

One of the best examples of the value of solid empirical data can be found in recent reviews of empirical studies related to the use of proxy consent for incompetent patients [12, 13]. These show fairly conclusively that some of the premises which have been used in ethical arguments for the use of family members as proxies are false. Few people have actually discussed severe illness and life-sustaining treatments with members of their family, and proxies are in general poor at predicting patients' preferences for life-sustaining treatments. Any argument building on assumptions about the ability of proxies to emulate the decisions of the patient must therefore be revised.

This example further illustrates another important feature of empirical ethics research. The research question asked has to be grounded in some kind of theoretical framework. The results on proxy decision-making mentioned above are only important in so far as we have a theory or a series of arguments which contain premises about proxy consent as 'substituted judgement'. If we argued for proxy consent purely on the basis of the close relationship between family members, another set of empirical data would be pertinent.

Teaching bioethics and promoting moral development

Most bioethicists teach students of various professions, lecture to professional or lay audiences, or write articles and books not aimed at their fellow bioethicists. They presumably do this for one or more of several reasons: because it is part of their job, because they are paid to do it, because it adds to their academic standing, or because they think it will benefit the audience and/or the future and present patients of the audience. If some of the motivation springs from a belief that affecting some change (moral development?) in the audience will be beneficial, then it seems that it would be of value to study whether such change occurs, and what teaching methods are most effective in bringing about change.

It is possible to find a number of studies in the medical literature which take this approach [14–20], and a recent book in nursing studies provides a valuable review of the available evidence [21]. It is clear from such works that teaching bioethics can bring about change in moral reasoning, recognition of moral problems, and moral actions; and there is evidence that some forms of teaching are more effective than others. Assessing whether the changes brought about in these studies are beneficial is a separate and controversial question, and the answer will vary widely depending on the underlying moral theory of the person doing the assessment.

In the actual teaching situation empirical ethics and ethics-related studies are also relevant. Knowledge about ethical attitudes and the mode of ethical thinking in the student population is important, so that one does not preach to the already converted, but concentrates on those areas were there is room for improvement, change, or clarification. When we teach 'harder' subjects like anatomy or biochemistry, we try to build on what the students already know, so that the level is neither too high nor too low. The same approach seems appropriate for bioethics.

Knowledge about the types of ethical problem that students are going to meet in their daily practice is also important in this context. The thought of teaching business ethics to MBA students by citing examples from the daily practice of a paediatrician strikes us as ludicrous, but is it not so ludicrous to teach medical ethics to medical students by using philosophical examples that are far removed from the daily clinical context. Teaching is often most successful when it engages the experiences of the students, and to do that we need to know what those experiences are. Fortunately, sociologists have furnished us with studies describing the life of medical students and young doctors, and we ought to take them into account. Two of the classics in this field are Howard Becker's *Boys in White – Student Culture in Medical School* [22] and Charles Bosk's *Forgive and Remember – Managing Medical Failure* [23] but there are also more recent studies available (see, for instance, [24–9]).

There are many problems with research that measures moral development or moral change, primarily because most of the instruments used to measure change come from one particular psychological/philosophical tradition – that is, the

Kohlberg tradition of cognitive-developmental theory, which views justice as the overriding moral concern. And, as it is well known from the Kohlberg–Gilligan debate reviewed in Chapter 1, not everyone accepts that the development of a more and more abstract conception of justice should count as moral progress [30, 31].

These problems are real and important, but they do not indicate that we should not try to measure the effect of our teaching. If one is not a Kohlbergian one will have to use or develop other instruments, such as the combined Kohlberg–Gilligan instrument developed by Self and Skeel [32].

Moral psychology

I now wish to move from the pragmatic to the metaethical use of empirical data in bioethics, and discuss the connection between moral psychology and ethical theory, since the former presents the most serious challenge to the view that no normative conclusions follow solely from empirical statements.

If we believe that 'ought implies can', and if the notion of possibility embedded in this 'can' is thicker than just 'not logically impossible', then it could matter normatively whether the thought patterns prescribed by a specific ethical theory could be performed by human beings. It is reasonable to assume that the 'can' in question must imply more than just logical possibility. There is no logical contradiction in the claim that 'Carl Lewis ought to jump over the Empire State Building to collect money for charity', and, given that the sum collected for charity if he managed to do so would undoubtedly be very large, he might actually have a moral obligation to do it. Most of us probably believe that Carl Lewis has no such obligation and should feel no moral compunction, because he cannot physically accomplish the feat, and this seems to indicate that human physical abilities play a role when we decide what obligations a human moral agent can have.

What, then, about human psychological traits? We have good reasons to believe that the human brain is not an all-purpose computer which can process whatever program it is given. Some simple functions which are hardwired in the brain (e.g., visual tracking) cannot be changed and other functions seem to be outside the range of most human beings (e.g. extracting the square root of two without paper and pencil). The same may well be true of some forms of ethical thought. It is, for instance, a common objection against any form of act-consequentialism requiring calculation of *all* consequences of a given act that no human being could perform these calculations. This indicates that we ought to adopt some version of Flanagan's Principle of Minimal Psychological Realism: 'Make sure when constructing a moral theory or projecting a moral ideal that the character, decision processing, and behavior prescribed are possible, or are perceived to be possible, for creatures like us' [33, p. 32]. An ethical theory that cannot conceivably be implemented on the computational hardware of the human brain, or which requires a kind of personality structure that cannot be attained by humans, is simply not an option for any human agent.

Such a theory could be put forward as an ideal with an acknowledgement that the ideal will never be instantiated in any human person. This would entail that it is impossible to lead a fully moral life. Such a consequence is not in itself enough to discredit the ideal. We have no guarantee that it is possible to live a fully moral life as a human being, and no guarantee that the demands of morality are not strenuous. But if it is the case that the ideal put forward is really inaccessible to humans, then we need a second order theory about what parts of the ideal we ought to strive for, and such a theory would have to take account of moral psychology, or would fall foul of the 'ought implies can' principle.

The crucial question, then, becomes whether empirical research can give us the knowledge we need. The promise of firm knowledge seems to be larger in those branches of psychology that are most intimately concerned with the hardware side of the human brain (that is, neuropsychology and cognitive science), whereas the possibility of getting firm knowledge about the range of possible motivational structures or the

limits of personality change seems more remote. It is, nevertheless, conceivable that the range of possible motivational
structures is constrained, and that this could be the object of
empirical research. For instance, it is not wholly unlikely that
the motivational structure advocated by a moral theory which
prescribed equal and non-trivial regard for every human (or
perhaps sentient?) being falls outside the possible range, and
that psychological studies could show this to be the case. We
may not presently know how much knowledge empirical studies will give, but we cannot *ex ante* assume that they will not
give any.

Conclusion

This chapter has argued for the conclusion that descriptive
ethics is of vital importance to normative bioethics, but what
is the proper relationship between these two subdisciplines? Is
it the case, as Hoffmaster has suggested, that ethnography
should save the life of medical ethics through a shift in
emphasis from theory-based to practice-based ethics [34]? As
Weaver and Trevino have pointed out there are at least three
possible ways of conceiving the relationship [35]: parallel, symbiotic, and integrative.

In a parallel relationship, normative and empirical ethics
are strictly separate fields each having its own set of theories,
and the only shared element is the area of interest (that is, certain kinds of behaviour). This is the view held by classical
social science, where moral categories like democracy or free-
dom are eschewed as value-laden [36].

A symbiotic relationship entails that there should be a col-
laborative relationship between normative and empirical
ethics. Each approach retains a distinct theoretical core, but
there is exchange of data and ideas, and each approach
acknowledges the contribution of the other to its own development.

Finally, an integrative relationship is the most far-reaching departure from the traditional divide between empirical
and normative ethics because it would entail the hybridisation

of the two approaches and the construction of a common theoretical core.

Most of the present chapter has argued that bioethics needs to establish a symbiotic relationship between its normative and empirical branch in order to move from the philosophers' ivory tower into the real world. Within bioethics this would in general entail that normative bioethicists would have to pay closer attention to the results of empirical studies, and perhaps even have to perform or initiate such studies themselves.

However, in the case of moral psychology a closer relationship is in order. This might not be an integrative relationship as conceived by Weaver and Trevino, since moral psychology would still only deliver a small part of the final normative product; but a relationship where the psychological constraints on human action are taken seriously, and where empirical data, and not just philosophical psychology, are used as the measure of these constraints. Moral psychology may not be sufficiently advanced to give definite answers to the questions asked [37], but perhaps this has more to do with the historically strained relationship between psychologists and moral philosophers than with the inherent possibilities in this field of study.

Notes

1 Consequences are to be understood in the broadest possible sense, i.e. as including the breach of strictly deontological principles.

2 In this and the following paragraphs the argument assumes a generally consequentialist moral theory. There seems to be almost universal agreement that consequences of actions actually do matter, apart from other right-making characteristics of actions. Very few would accept the dictum 'Fiat justitia, pereat mundus'. But even on a strict deontological theory a parallel argument could be produced. If, for instance, we accept the principle 'Do not betray the trust of others', it is obvious that we need to know what others trust us to do if we live in a morally pluralistic society and want to apply the principle.

3 Given that all accept the set of moral rules, their motivation for acting against them must be outside the area of morality.

References

1 Nicholson, R., Empirical data is vital to bioethics. *Bulletin of Medical Ethics* 1993; 86 (March): 16–24.

2 Braddock, H., The role of empirical research in medical ethics: asking questions or answering them? *The Journal of Clinical Ethics* 1994; 5: 144–7.

3 Stolman, Cynthia J., Should medical encounters be studied using ethnographic techniques? *The Journal of Clinical Ethics* 1993; 4: 183–5.

4 Beauchamp, T. L., Childress, J. F., *The Principles of Biomedical Ethics* (4th edn). Oxford: Oxford University Press, 1994.

5 Sidgwick, H., *The Methods of Ethics* (7th edn). London: Macmillan and Company, 1907.

6 Siegler, M., Pellegrino, E. D., Singer, P. A., Clinical medical ethics. *The Journal of Clinical Ethics* 1991; 1: 5–9.

7 Kerrigan, D. D., Thevasagayam, R. S., Woods, T. O., McWelch, I., Thomas, W. E., Shorthouse, A. J., Dennison, A. R., Who's afraid of informed consent? *BMJ* 1993; 306: 298–300.

8 Appelbaum, P. S., Kapen, G., Walters, B., Lidz, C., Roth, L. H., Confidentiality: an empirical test of the utilitarian perspective. *Bulletin of the American Academy of Psychiatry and Law* 1984; 12: 109–16.

9 Caplan, A. L., Can applied ethics be effective in health care and should it strive to be? In: Ackerman, T. F., Graber, G. C., Reynolds, C. H., Thomasma, D. C. (eds), *Clinical Medical Ethics – Exploration and Assessment*. Lanham, MD: University Press of America, 1987: pp. 131–43.

10 Dewey, J., Tufts, J., *Ethics*. New York: Henry Holt and Co., 1908.

11 Brody, B. A., Assessing empirical research in bioethics. *Theoretical Medicine* 1993; 14: 211–19.

12 Emanuel, E. J., Emanuel, L. L., Proxy decision making for incompetent patients – an ethical and empirical analysis. *JAMA* 1992; 267: 2067–71.

13 Pearlman, R. A., Miles, S. H., Arnold, R. M., Contributions of empirical research to medical ethics. *Theoretical Medicine* 1993; 14: 197–210.

14 Mitchell, K. R., Myser, C., Kerridge, I. H., Assessing the clinical ethical competence of undergraduate medical students. *Journal of Medical Ethics* 1993; 19: 230–6.

15 Siegler, M., Rezler, A. G., Connell. K. J., Using simulated case studies to evaluate a clinical ethics course for junior students. *Journal of Medical Education* 1982; 57: 380–5.

16 Self, D. J., Wolinsky, F. D., Baldwin, D. C., The effect of teaching medical ethics on medical students' moral reasoning. *Academic Medicine* 1989; 64: 755–9.

17 Self, D. J., Baldwin, D. C., Wolinsky, F. D., Evaluation of teaching med-

ical ethics by an assessment of moral reasoning. *Medical Education* 1992; 26: 178–84.

18 Self, D. J., Schrader, D.E., Baldwin, D. C., Wolinsky, F. D., The moral development of medical students: a pilot study of the possible influence of medical education. *Medical Education* 1993; 27: 26–34.

19 Self, D. J., Baldwin, D. C., Olivarez, M., Teaching medical ethics to first-year students by using film discussion to develop their moral reasoning. *Academic Medicine* 1993; 68: 383–5.

20 Stevens, N. G., McCormick, T. R., What are students thinking when we present ethics cases?: an example focusing on confidentiality and substance abuse. *Journal of Medical Ethics* 1994; 20: 112–17.

21 Silva, M. C., Sorrell, J. M., *Research on Ethics in Nursing Education: An Integrative Review and Critique.* New York: National League for Nursing Press, 1991.

22 Becker, H. S., Geer, B., Hughes, E. C., Strauss, A. L., *Boys in White – Student Culture in Medical School.* Chicago: University of Chicago Press, 1961.

23 Bosk, C. L., *Forgive and Remember – Managing Medical Failure.* Chicago: University of Chicago Press, 1979.

24 Baldwin, D. C., Daugherty, S. R., Rowley, B. D., Schwarz, M. D., Cheating in medical school: a survey of Second-year students at 31 schools. *Academic Medicine* 1996; 71: 267–73.

25 Hays, L. R., Cheever, T., Patel, P., Medical student suicide, 1989–1994. *American Journal of Psychiatry* 1996; 153: 553–5.

26 Merril, J. M., Laux, L.F., Lorimor, R.J., Thornby, J. L., Vallbona, C., Measuring social desirability among senior medical students. *Psychological Reports* 1995; 77(3, pt 1): 859–64.

27 Bissonnette, R., O'Shea, R.M., Horwitz, M., Route, C. F., A data-generated basis for medical ethics education: categorizing issues experienced by students during clinical training. *Academic Medicine* 1995; 70: 1035–7.

28 Wolf, T. M., Heller, S. S., Camp, C. J., Faucett, J. M., The process of coping with a gross anatomy exam during the first year of medical school. *British Journal of Medical Psychology* 1995; 68(pt 1): 85–7.

29 Feudtner, C., Christakis, D. A., Christakis, N. A., Do clinical clerks suffer ethical erosion? students' perceptions of their ethical environment and personal development. *Academic Medicine* 1994; 69: 670–9.

30 Gilligan, C., *In a Different Voice: Psychological Theory and Women's Development.* Cambridge, MA: Harvard University Press, 1982.

31 Kohlberg, L., *The Philosophy of Moral Development.* New York: Harper and Row, 1981.

32 Self, D. J., Skeel, J. D., Facilitating healthcare ethics research: assessment of moral reasoning and moral orientation from a single interview. *Cambridge Quarterly of Health Care Ethics* 1992; 1: 371–6.

33 Flanagan, O., *Varieties of Moral Personality – Ethics and Psychological Realism*. Cambridge, MA.: Harvard University Press, 1991.

34 Hoffmaster, B., Can ethnography save the life of medical ethics. *Social Science and Medicine* 1992; 35: 1421–31.

35 Weaver, G. R., Trevino, L. K., Normative and empirical business ethics: separation, marriage of convenience, or marriage of necessity. *Business Ethics Quarterly* 1994; 4: 129–43.

36 Kerlinger, F. N., *Foundations of Behavioral Research*. New York: Holt, Rinehart and Winston, 1986.

37 Waterman, A. S., On the uses of psychological theory and research in the process of ethical inquiry. *Psychological Bulletin* 1988; 103(3): 283–98.

3

The scientific status of qualitative research

Yet when we follow their most proper intention, in all the sciences we relate ourselves to beings themselves. Precisely from the point of view of the sciences or disciplines no field takes precedence over another, neither nature over history nor vice versa. No particular way of treating objects of inquiry dominates the others. Mathematical knowledge is no more rigorous than philological-historical knowledge. It merely has the character of 'exactness', which does not coincide with rigor. To demand exactness in the study of history is to violate the idea of the specific rigor of the humanities. [1, p. 94]

Introduction

Within health care research, qualitative research is still regarded as unscientific by many scientists. When the Danish Medical Association put forward a proposal for a research policy in the summer of 1995 [2], the section that led to the largest debate called for support for humanistic research in health care. A neuroanatomist commented from the podium that he was very sceptical about this section. He believed that all his own research was humanistic, and he did not feel certain that the humanities could actually claim to possess anything worthy of the name 'scientific methods' [3].

The empirical part of this book utilises qualitative methods, and it is therefore of obvious importance to the present project to analyse the scientific status of qualitative research. But such an analysis is also of interest in other contexts.

It is evident that to call an activity scientific is to make a claim with great rhetorical power in the public debate. Scientific activity is connected to institutions with great public prestige (e.g., universities), and the state supports scientific studies in most countries. To be able to claim scientific status is thus important in debates on resource allocation.

It is also clear that claims to possess independent knowledge play a large role in the development towards professionalisation of various groups within the health care sector. The development of nursing science has, for instance, been part of a deliberate strategy aiming at transforming nurses from being the handmaidens of the physicians to being professionals with independent responsibility.

Choice of strategy

Proponents of qualitative research can pursue two different strategies in discussions about its scientific status. The first strategy is to concentrate on an attack on quantitative research in order to show that it is less scientifically rigorous than is generally believed, the claim being that the arguments put forward against qualitative research affect the scientific status of quantitative research just as much (or more). The second strategy is to concentrate effort on showing that qualitative research can fulfil the criteria for scientific status just as well as quantitative research can. It is this second strategy that I will try to pursue here. The old adage may well claim that the best defence is attack, but attacking quantitative research and claiming that it is unscientific is not likely to lead to any improvement of the communication between qualitative and quantitative researchers.

My aim in this chapter is to present an account of the scientific status of qualitative research which builds on premises that the 'average' health care professional can accept. I think that such an account is necessary if the results of qualitative studies are to gain currency in scientific discourse and influence medical decision-making. My philosophical project in this chapter is thus connected with the approach followed by Tschudi [4], but is antithetical to the approaches of qualitative theorists such as Polkinghorne or Kvale [5, 6].

The separate paradigm idea

This choice of strategy also leads me to reject accounts of qualitative research that try to establish its scientific status by positing a separate hermeneutic, phenomenological, interpretative, or qualitative research paradigm in the Kuhnian sense [7, 8]. I agree with Lunde that there is no reason to believe that the main paradigm of medical research is going to be replaced, and with her conclusion that the main task is to change components of this paradigm, not to overthrow it [9]. Even if we do not take Kuhn's initial claim of radical incommensurability between paradigms seriously, positing two separate paradigms, a qualitative and a quantitative, still creates at least three kinds of problem.

First, there is the problem that if the concept of research paradigm is understood as the basic implicit and explicit assumptions underlying a specific research programme, then it is difficult to see how one person could hold more than one paradigm at the same time without being involved in blatant inconsistency (if the two paradigms are substantially different). If one paradigm claims that subjectivity is an important positive factor in the research process, and the other claims that it is a negative factor, then holding both paradigms will be inconsistent. This implies that the two paradigms cannot be complementary, but only parallel. A person could try to pursue research within both paradigms, but he or she would then have to bracket off all or part of one paradigm when working within the other, and would in this way be engaged in performative inconsistency.

The second problem follows from the first. If the two paradigms cannot be held simultaneously, and if they delimit the field of true science differently, then it follows by necessity that holders of the paradigms will be in disagreement about the status of some areas of research practice, and that this disagreement is insoluble because it follows directly from core features in the two paradigms. That is, even if there is no incommensurability, there may still be conflict about whether something is truly a scientific enterprise.

Third, this disagreement will in itself create a second order communication problem. Findings originating from research in the disputed area will only be acceptable as scientific within one of the paradigms, and will be rejected by holders of the other paradigm. To have your research declared non-scientific is not taken lightly by most researchers, and it is likely that such a statement will lead to the rapid cessation of communication.

Adherence to a separate qualitative paradigm is therefore likely to lead to problems in communications amongst the large majority of health care professionals who still hold a primarily quantitative paradigm. This conclusion is reinforced by the experiences from work in research groups with internal paradigmatic differences summarised by Launsø and Rieper [10].

This practical communication problem is going to be especially problematic if the qualitative paradigm includes a rejection of a correspondence theory of truth.[1] Some qualitative theorists want to move to a pragmatic theory of truth,[2] because they connect positivism and the correspondence theory of truth, and claim that the latter is antithetical to the assumptions of human science research [13]. At this point, real paradigmatic incommensurability threatens, because scientific communication and argument are dependent on a common understanding of what statements count as true or valid.

It is also questionable whether it is the case that there is really only one qualitative paradigm. The philosophies underlying, say, grounded theory (see p. 82) and Heideggerian hermeneutic phenomenology are so different that it is difficult to see that these two qualitative research traditions can be accommodated within the same paradigm. If this is true, it has unfortunate consequences: namely, that Leininger's assertion that 'one cannot mix research methods across qualitative and quantitative paradigms, but one can mix methods within each paradigm' [8, p. 101] is false, and that there is great scope for internecine strife in the qualitative camp.

Qualitative and quantitative

I have consistently used the terms qualitative and quantitative research here, but this is only for lack of better terms. The common use of the qualitative/quantitative distinction points to two rather distinct approaches to science, but the two labels are highly misleading in several ways.

There is no sharp distinction between qualitative and quantitative data. Some data may be easier to quantify than others, but there are none that are inherently quantitative. If, for instance, we look at height, we find that it is easily quantifiable, but it can also be classified by the qualitative predicates 'tall', 'small', 'giant', 'dwarf', etc. The same holds the other way around. Although some data may be very difficult to quantify, there are no inherently qualitative data. Even mental states may be quantifiable if some form of type-type identity holds for the relationship between brain and mental events [14].

The failure of the qualitative/quantitative distinction with regard to data is perhaps best illustrated by a Danish book with the promising title *Analyse af Kvalitative Data – En Grundbog for Samfundsvidenskaberne* (*Analysis of Qualitative Data – A Primer for the Social Sciences*) [15]. The subject matter of the book is the statistical analysis of data from questionnaires in those cases where the answers are categorical and do not fall into any kind of natural ranking. Such data are obviously qualitative in the sense that they are difficult to scale, but as the application of the methods in the book show, they could as easily be called quantitative, because they are easy to enumerate and can be analysed by applying numerical methods.

On the level of analysis the distinction is not sharp either. Quantification can be of great use in qualitative research (e.g. many of the diagrams in Miles's and Huberman's *Qualitative Data Analysis* build on implicit quantification [16]), and many forms of quantitative research incorporate large elements of interpretation in their research procedures.

The really important distinction seems to me, instead, to turn on the role of interpretation in the research process, and the relationship between quantification and interpretation. What mainly distinguishes the cluster of procedures called 'qualitative research' from that called 'quantitative research' is that the latter tries to reduce the role of interpretation in all the phases of the research process except the last, where the results are interpreted and put in perspective in the traditional 'discussion' section of scientific papers. In contrast to this, the qualitative researcher often relies explicitly on interpretation in all phases of the research process, from the collection of data to the final discussion. A better terminology would therefore be a distinction between interpretative and non-interpretative forms of research, but the terms qualitative and quantitative are so entrenched that they will be hard to get rid of. I have, therefore, resigned myself to continue using them here.

Phenomenology and hermeneutics

A common way of arguing for the scientific validity of qualitative research is to adopt either a phenomenological approach, following Husserl, Merleau-Ponty, or Levinas, or an existentialist approach, following Heidegger or Sartre [17–19]. I do not think that this is a very fruitful strategy. The philosophy is difficult to understand, even for professional philosophers, and although Husserl envisioned his phenomenology as the foundation of a new science [20], the other philosophers mentioned here either explicitly rejected aspirations towards a philosophy of science, or simply did not pursue any extension of their philosophy to include a philosophy of science.

If a philosophy of science could be developed from phenomenology or existentialism, it would be very different from the mainstream of philosophy of science, and would truly constitute a new paradigm in Kuhn's sense. It is, for instance, difficult to see how a radical phenomenological and a Popperian philosopher of science could even begin to communicate.

The only serious attempt to develop concurrently a philosophy of science and a research methodology on a phenomenological basis is ethnomethodology which was developed by Garfinkel, and built upon the philosophy of science elaborated by Schutz, who was a pupil of Husserl [21, 22]. In the literature it is evident that this grounding in a different philosophy also leads to a rather different kind of science.

Since one of my aims is to develop an account of the scientific status of qualitative science which is understandable to the 'average' health care professional an end result of radical incommensurability is obviously undesirable. I will therefore not pursue the phenomenological and existentialist approaches further here.

Social constructivism and constructionism

I shall also leave out a detailed discussion of social constructivism and social constructionism. Social constructionism is, however, in rapid ascendence as a philosophy of social science, which makes it necessary to say at least a few words about this school of thought.

A radical social constructionist approach would simply make any kind of research involving data collection from respondents superfluous. Because the world is constructed through language, and language is constructed socially, we only have to look at the meaning of the words; there is no need for further data. The consequences of this view are probably best exemplified by presenting some quotes from a paper by Gergen and Gergen which have quickly become notorious. They write:

> Within a social constructionist framework, we locate new vistas for solving the problem of origins. More specifically, we abandon the problem of the origin of ideas within the head, and shift concern to the emergence of language within communities.
>
> [...]
>
> In this sense, scientists approach their problems with a range of linguistic predispositions already at hand. For them to generate understanding is to apply the existing language to the problem at hand.
>
> [...]
>
> Consider, for example, the theorist who wishes to 'understand' the nature of jealousy. By theoretical understanding generally the scientific establishment means the production of a series of propositions of the 'if ... then' variety. These propositions should describe the central features of the 'phenomenon'. For the constructionist,

however, jealousy is not a feature of the world independent of a language system. Instead, 'jealousy' is a linguistic integer enmeshed in cultural codes of communicating (and acting). Whether or not one uses the term 'jealousy' does not depend on what is 'actually the case', but on local conventions of naming or indexing patterns of events. By the same token, the 'determinants' or 'antecedents' of jealousy are not read from nature, nor derived logically from observation. They, too, are constituents of an elaborate code of intelligibility. [23, pp. 80–1]

The authors then analyse the linguistic meaning of jealousy and go on to present the following comments:

Combining the above formulation, one can thus derive the proposition:

4. People who are low in self-esteem will be more highly prone to jealousy than those who are high in self-esteem.

This last proposition enables the investigator to move from the simple level of definition and homily to something on the order of a 'theoretical insight' with important practical implications for inter-personal relationships. It must be realised, however, that the entire formulation is based on an elaboration of definitions already embedded within the cultural code. Such propositions stand intelligible without a single observation of persons in action.

[...]

The confirmations (or disconfirmations) of hypotheses through research findings are achieved through social consensus, not through observation of the 'facts'. The 'empirical test' is possible because the conventions of linguistic indexing are so fully shared ('so commonsensical') that they appear to 'reflect' reality. Thus, for example, we can treat the proposition 'John was in class this morning' as empirically verifiable because the meaning of the terms of the proposition are so broadly shared that they seem to be 'mirrors' of the world.

[...]

Thus, whether or not John was *actually* in class depends on what one is willing to call 'John', 'class', 'in' and the like and not on what is given to observation. [23, pp. 81–2, emphasis in the original]

As an exemplification of social constructionist thought, these quotes provide ample evidence that the constructionist project is built on extremely questionable assumptions about the connection between language and reality, and on faulty reasoning.

It is true that the meaning of the sentence 'John was in class this morning', and its empirical verifiability, to some extent depend on the meaning of the six individual words in the sentence, but from this it does not follow that whether John was actually in class *only* depends on these linguistic facts. Even if I am a fully competent member of your linguistic community, I could (in most circumstances) not answer the question 'Was John in class this morning?' without having access to some observational data. Gergen and Gergen invalidly infer the conclusion 'x is *only* dependent on y' from the premise 'x is dependent on y'.

Gergen and Gergen also totally disregard the many instances in the history of science in which propositions derived by theoretical analysis have been disconfirmed by empirical observation. Their proposition about the connection between jealousy and self-esteem may well be 'intelligible without a single observation of persons in action', but intelligibility and epistemic warrant are not the same. The sentence 'the moon is made of grey-blue cheese' is fully intelligible, but is has no epistemic warrant whatsoever (and empirical observation shows that it is actually false). Intelligibility is simply not sufficient to ground a claim to possess knowledge, and anybody who tried to live their life based on 'knowledge' gained by social constructionist analysis would soon realise that there is an unforgiving external world ready to 'punish' those who do not take adequate account of reality.

Less radical versions of social constructivism make more sense, but to me the whole approach seems to be more suitable for history and sociology of science than for philosophy of science. We know, for instance, that disease concepts and images of particular diseases are socially constructed and differ from country to country [24, 25]. We also know that these different constructions are created by intricate social processes, and not by pure rational deliberation. But what are the implications of these findings for philosophy of science? Bruno Latour describes the construction of the disease anthrax as part of the 'Pasteurisation of France', but it seems safe to assume that people and animals died of anthrax in France even before Pasteur identified/constructed *Bacillus anthracis* as the causative agent. It is also difficult to imagine that some other scientist would not have found the bacterium and constructed the disease at some later point if Pasteur had missed it. Such a later construction could well have been different in some ways, but how large the difference could have been is an open question. And the structure of the external world would in all cases set some limitations for the possible constructions.

Social constructivism is important for philosophy of science because its critique of traditional sociology of science dispels the naive picture of the scientist involved in a purely rational search for knowledge. But it has little to offer in terms of a positive account of science.

Habermas and emancipatory social research

Another important philosophical school which has been connected with qualitative research is the later Frankfurt school and its main figure Jürgen Habermas [26–8]. There has been great interest in his ideas about the encroachment of the system-world on the life-world, about communication without domination as a regulative ideal for human interaction, and about a division of the sciences according to the main interests behind the scientific endeavour (technical, practical, emancipatory). Much of what is called 'action research' is built on Habermasian ideas [29].

It is, however, difficult to see how a Habermasian approach can provide a full justification for qualitative research as it is presently carried out. One could start with taking communication without domination as the regulative ideal for the data-collection process and perhaps even for the planning stage of research projects. This would probably lead to methodological guidelines that were somewhat different from those advocated by qualitative methodologists today (e.g., ordinary interviewing might not be appropriate because it requires or generates an unequal distribution of power), but the final research practice would still be recognisable as qualitative research. There

is, however, one remaining problem. Even if new methodological guidelines were to be followed, it would not in and of
itself guarantee that the research would be emancipatory.
Qualitative researchers can be driven by all three kinds of
research interest, and may in some cases actually contribute to
the expansion of the system-world. The methodology does not
in itself preclude such an outcome. Even if a research project
were to be carried out with Habermasian methodology, we
would still have to judge what kind of research interest this
specific project embodied.

A Habermasian approach can therefore be valuable in
developing qualitative methodology and in assessing research
practice from a political and moral point of view, but it does
not offer an easy way to scientific legitimation of all qualitative research in one fell swoop.

Delimiting the field

Even a cursory glance at the literature makes it obvious that
the field of qualitative research is very broad, ranging from
historical studies and single case-studies to large multi-centre,
multi-author studies with rigorous interview guides and professional interviewers. It is unlikely that it will be possible to
find one single set of arguments that will give scientific status
to all of these quite disparate research procedures.

I will therefore concentrate on qualitative research with
the following characteristics:

1. data are collected by contact with respondents in the field
    of interest (e.g. by means of interviews, focus groups, or
    observation);
2. the data collection is based on a specific statement of the
    main research questions, which have been developed based
    on some knowledge of the extant literature;
3. the aim of the data analysis is to generate public knowl-
    edge through the use of some publicly describable method.

In short, the arguments presented here will presuppose direct
gathering of data, a knowledgeable researcher, and some pub-

licly describable method. I am not claiming that a research
project that lacks one or more of these three characteristics
cannot be scientific, but only that the arguments presented in
the following will only pertain to research having these characteristics.

Some classic forms of qualitative research do fall outside
these limitations (e.g., many classical ethnographies of 'primi-
tive people'). I think that arguments can be produced in favour
of the scientific status of these forms of qualitative research,
but it is a task which falls outside the scope of this chapter.

I do not think, however, that it is possible to mount any
defence for the suggestion sometimes heard that the researcher
should approach the field without any preconceptions and
without any study of the literature. This methodological advice
is naive and dangerous. It disregards the fact that our access to
data is never unmediated. Perception is always theory-laden
(or always from a certain horizon of understanding), and there
is no reason to believe that the implicit theories influencing
our 'normal' everyday perception of events have any advantages over a reflectively accepted scientific theory. Believing
that one can be in an epistemological *status nascendi* with a
mind as open and untainted as the *tabula rasa* of the early
British empiricists can only create a blind spot [30], making it
impossible even to begin to identify the theoretical presuppo-
sitions in one's work.

What is science?

In order to be able to decide whether something constitutes a
valid scientific enterprise it is necessary first to decide how one
could go about answering that question, or, in a more technical sense, how one should find a demarcation criterion that is
able to distinguish science from non-science.

One possibility is to list all those enterprises we presently
regard as scientific and then try to elucidate what they have
in common. I will not carry out that exercise here, but I am
fairly certain that the answer will be 'nothing'. There is nothing that all enterprises labelled as science have in common,

unless we allow fuzzy characteristics such as 'having a critical attitude towards your own theories'. This failure to find some common characteristic has led critics of the status of science (most notably Feyerabend) to conclude that science is just a rhetorical term [31]. This is, however, a much too far-reaching conclusion. If we take Wittgenstein's famous example of the impossibility of defining 'chair', it does not show that chairs do not exist, it only shows that there is not one thing which all chairs have in common, which is exclusive to chairs, and which defines 'chairness'.

The other possible way to answer the quest for a demarcation criterion between science and non-science is to try to decide on a normative criterion – that is, one that stipulates some condition which an enterprise must fulfil in order to count as science. Choosing this option may lead to a situation where some enterprises must be relabelled. Some of the things we now call science may not fulfil the criterion, and some things not presently recognised as sciences may fulfil it. This is the approach chosen by the positivists, and later by Popper and Lakatos.

For the logical positivists in the Vienna circle, the demarcation criterion was verification. Only sentences that could be verified against sense data were seen as meaningful, and only such sentences could form the basis for scientific knowledge.

Positivism

At this point I should like to exorcise the ghost of positivism from the debate about the scientific status of qualitative research. As a philosophy of science, positivism has been dead for decades, and the verification criterion supposed to distinguish between meaningful and non-meaningful statements was exposed as self-referential (and thereby meaningless for the positivist himself) by Popper in 1934 in his *Logik der Forschung* (that is, more than sixty years ago) [32]. It is therefore a waste of energy to continue to fight against positivism, and to direct one's arguments against this position, as if it were still a valid contender for a normative philosophy of science; and it is directly misleading to label opponents of qualitative research as positivists if this is intended to describe their philosophy of science. Many opponents of qualitative research are actually Popperian falsificationists, and their opposition is directly related to a claim that the interpretative approach of qualitative research is just some non-stringent form of inductive verification in disguise.

To dichotomise the world of science in positivism on the one hand and interpretative science on the other can in the end only obscure the problems by establishing a convenient straw man. But, unfortunately, it is a practice that is fairly widespread, especially in nursing science and in sociology and psychology. A particularly clear example can be found in a table taken from an advanced book on nursing science (see Table 3.1, redrawn from [33, p. 29]). In the discourse where this table appears it is not necessary to explain that qualitative methods must be good, since they are on the side where all the positive words have been placed. Who in their right mind would ever prefer 'persistence' to 'change' or, horror of horrors, 'positivism' to 'feminism'?

Table 3.1   Views of science

Paradigm I: *Received view of science*	Paradigm II: *Perceived view of science*
empiricism	historicism
positivism	feminism
persistence	change
mechanism	organicism
facts ahistorical	facts historical
facts acontextual	facts contextual
quantitative methods	qualitative methods

It may well be true that many health care professionals are still crypto-positivist. But to claim that they hold positivism as a philosophy of science is about as philosophically illuminating and important as the claim that most people hold a generative theory of causality (that is, that the cause generates the consequence). Both statements may be empirically true, but only if the meaning of the term theory is stretched to encompass any set of beliefs about a given subject (even sets of belief that have never been rationally scrutinised by the person holding the beliefs). All health care professionals I have met can easily be brought to understand why positivism is false as a philosophy of science (that is, they can understand the induction problem and the self-referential nature of verificationism when it is explained to them). But even when they have been 'converted' from positivism to Popperian falsificationism, many still believe that qualitative research is not proper science. This belief is therefore not only based on crypto-positivism, it must represent some other problem as well.

If we are to elucidate this problem and present arguments for the scientific status of qualitative research, it is singularly unhelpful to continue to use the blanket term 'positivist' for all opponents of qualitative research.

Falsification and research programmes

The main figure in classical philosophy of science is Karl Popper, who put forward in his work a demarcation criterion, and a number of important ideas about other problems in the philosophy of science (for an account of the philosophy of science prior to Popper, see Losee [34]). Because of Popper's influence, many later philosophers of science have positioned themselves in full or partial opposition to his ideas. It is therefore worthwhile to present a short summary of these ideas.

Popper's demarcation criterion is falsifiability. A theory is a scientific theory if it can be falsified by experiment or simple observation. Science should therefore progress by proposing bold hypotheses, testing them, and discarding those that are falsified. A hypothesis or theory can never be proven,[3] but, as it withstands sustained attempts of falsification, it becomes more and more corroborated. For Popper, corroboration is not a species of induction, but basically a comparative instrument when theories are compared:

> By the degree of corroboration of a theory I mean a concise report evaluating the state (at a certain time t) of the critical discussion of

a theory, with respect to the way it solves its problems; its degree of testability; the severity of the tests it has undergone; and the way it has stood up to these tests. Corroboration (or degree of corroboration) is thus an evaluating *report of past performance*. Like preference, it is essentially comparative: in general, one can only say that the theory A has a higher (or lower) degree of corroboration than a competing theory B, in the light of the critical discussion, which includes testing, *up to some time t*. [35, p. 18, emphasis in original]

Popper also argued that we have no immediate access to the external world because all observations are theory-laden. What I see depends on my theories about the world (theories here taken in a broad sense). Finally, he made a distinction between the 'context of discovery' where hypotheses are generated, and the 'context of justification' where they are tested. He believed that normative rules for the conduct of scientists were appropriate in the context of justification, but that the processes in the context of discovery lay mostly outside the realm of philosophy of science.

A common way to try to fit qualitative research into this framework has been to relegate qualitative research to a role solely in the context of discovery. First you do qualitative research to develop new ideas, and then you test these ideas with rigorous quantitative methods (this model has been the traditional model in quantitative sociology). But this approach is not satisfactory seen from the point of view of the qualitative researcher. Most qualitative researchers believe that part (or all) of their research can stand alone as producing valid scientific knowledge, without necessarily having to be tested by quantitative methods — that is, qualitative research is also claimed to be a valid method in the context of justification. It is important to note that this does not involve a claim that scientific knowledge gained through qualitative research should never be questioned and never tested in new situations. The claim is only that this kind of scientific knowledge should be awarded the same, necessarily provisional status as scientific knowledge gained through quantitative research.

One problem with Popper's philosophy of science and his demarcation criterion is that hypotheses do not occur in isolation. In any given experimental situation there is an infinite number of assumptions at play, and a given falsifying experimental result can be interpreted as falsifying a number of these different hypotheses (the Quine–Duhem problem). This was stated by Quine as the following three propositions:

1. It is misleading to speak of the 'empirical content' of an individual statement;
2. any statement can be retained as true provided that sufficiently drastic adjustments are made elsewhere in the system; and
3. there is no sharp boundary between synthetic statements whose truth (or falsity) is contingent upon empirical evidence, and analytic statements whose truth (or falsity) is independent of empirical evidence. [36, p. 43]

This critique, combined with Kuhn's ideas about paradigms and the historical development of science, led Imre Lakatos to propose a reformulation of the Popperian approach, shifting the emphasis from individual hypotheses to whole research programmes [37]. According to Lakatos, a given research programme consists of four components: a hard core of basic assumptions, a set of auxilliary hypotheses, a negative heuristic specifying paths of research to avoid, and a positive heuristic specifying paths of research to pursue. The hard core contains those assumptions that are central to the research programme, and which the scientists within the programme are not willing to discard. These assumptions are deemed irrefutable. Any apparent falsification of an assumption in the hard core will be interpreted as a falsification of one or more of the auxiliary hypotheses within the protective belt around the hard core.

A research programme is evaluated through the series of successive theories that are generated by the positive heuristic. A research programme is progressive as long as it is true of the series of theories T_1–T_n that:

1. T_n accounts for the previous successes of T_{n-1};
2. T_n has greater empirical content than T_{n-1}; and
3. Some of the excess content of T_n has been corroborated. [34, p. 231]

A research program for which this is not true is said to be degenerating. One common symptom of a degenerating research programme is the invention of immunising or *ad hoc* assumptions which are brought in when the data contradict the theory. According to Lakatos, the question of whether or not a scientist should leave a degenerating programme cannot be answered with any certainty, partly because it depends on the history of the programme and the availability of other progressive programmes [37].

Chalmers has developed Lakatos's idea, and has proposed an evolutionary account explaining why degenerating programmes will, in the end, cease to exist. He argues that research funding and young scientists will move toward research programmes that are progressive and generate interesting new findings – a process of 'natural selection' that will select against research programmes that are degenerate for longer periods of time [38].

Is there any way to fit qualitative research into this normative framework?

First of all, it is important to note that there are no arguments available to support the contention that qualitative research does not generate knowledge. If we accept the classical tripartite definition of knowledge first discussed by Plato, where knowledge is defined as true, justified belief [39, 40], there can be no doubt that some of the findings generated by qualitative research constitute knowledge in the commonly used sense of that word. This conclusion also holds for the new proposals for a definition of knowledge put forward following the publication of the Gettier examples, which showed that there were inherent problems in the old tripartite definition [41, 42]. What is at stake is the further claim that qualitative research can generate scientific knowledge.

To assess that claim it is necessary to look more closely at the methods employed in qualitative research. This raises the problem that few qualitative methodologies are fully described in the available literature, and that the number of methodologies 'on the market' is very large. What I have to say in the

following will therefore necessarily have to build on a somewhat stylised account of those qualitative research methodologies which share the three characteristics outlined above – that
is, primary data collection, specific research questions, and the
aim of producing public knowledge.

If we simplify the research process to the greatest possible
extent, we get the following scheme:

research question → data collection → analysis → scientific knowledge

But reality is usually more complex. The research question
may change over time, data collection and analysis may be
occurring simultaneously, and the final product – scientific
knowledge – may be generated piecemeal and over long periods of time. The picture shown in Figure 3.1 is therefore a
more faithful account of the process.

Figure 3.1 Research process

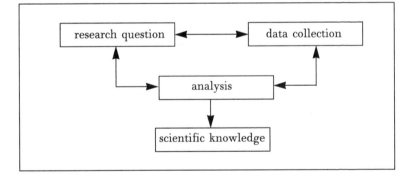

If we move back for a moment to the more simplified
scheme it becomes clear that the scientific status of qualitative
research depends mainly on the internal logic of the analytic
method. There are also certain conditions that must be fulfilled regarding data collection methods, but these will mainly
influence the possibility of generalising the findings.

But what, then, is the analytic logic of qualitative methodology? On this point the methodological literature is fairly vague,

and the actual suggestions regarding concrete methodology and contradictory, as can be seen from the following extracts:

Concepts are the basic building blocks of theory. Open coding in grounded theory method is the analytic process by which concepts are identified and developed in terms of their properties and dimensions. The basic analytic procedures by which this is accomplished are: the asking of questions about the data; and the making of comparisons for similarities and differences between each incident, event, and other instances of phenomena. Similar events and incidents are labeled and grouped to form categories. [43, p. 74]

Axial coding is the process of relating subcategories to a category. It is a complex process of inductive and deductive thinking involving several steps. [43, p. 114]

Through an ongoing process of data collection and analysis, the researcher is involved in a cycle of inductive and deductive reasoning until sufficient data have been reviewed to arrive at a dense theoretical explanation. [44, p. 175]

Sauer describes the overwhelming process of analyzing the dialogues and separating out themes for each informant. With themes identified for each informant, variations in themes could be selected out. ... For example, the identification of a conceptual category of 'planned, orderly lives', was advanced as one of the ground structures of the lived experiences of delayed parenthood for women. ... The meaningfulness of transition to delayed parenthood becomes more comprehensible when viewed from this conceptual framework of 'planned, orderly lives'. [45, p. 170]

The above progression illustrates the circular movement of hermeneutic research from understanding to interpretation to deeper understanding to more comprehensive interpretation. After immersing myself in the residents' lives (understanding), I began to analyze my notes and interviews (interpretation) to make sense out of them. My flash of (deeper understanding of) how surviving played such a central role for them led me to reanalyze my transcripts, diagrams, and models in light of the centrality of surviving (more comprehensive interpretation). Following this, I returned to observe and interview the residents (aiming for greater understanding and even further development of the interpretive account). Thus, as I moved around the hermeneutic circle, my understanding continued to deepen and my account became more coherent, cohesive, and comprehensive. [46, p. 119].

It is clear that the analytic logic prescribed by qualitative methodologists is neither straightforwardly inductive (the analysis is not only aimed at amassing evidence), nor hypothetico-deductive in the Hempelian sense of seeking a covering law explanation. What is prescribed, and, perhaps even more important, what qualitative researchers do, is look for an inference to the best explanation – that is, the account that is best able to make sense of the data. This indicates that the analytic logic is essentially abductive.

Peirce, abduction, and coherence

The idea of abduction as a valid mode of inference is closely connected with the philosophy of the American pragmatist philosopher C. S. Peirce. Peirce developed his ideas about abduction over a long period of time, and used at least three different names for this mode of inference: hypothesis, abduction, and retroduction [47]. He maintained that abduction was actually the basic inference, because he saw all perception as involving abduction. Our sensory experience of percepts is vague, and it is by a process of abduction that they become definite perceptions (an idea that is similar to Popper's insistence on the influence of theory on perception). Peirce's first 'canonical' statement of the difference between abduction (hypothesis) and induction reads as follows:

> By induction, we conclude that facts, similar to observed facts, are true in cases not examined. By hypothesis, we conclude the existence of a fact quite different from anything observed, from which, according to known laws, something observed would necessarily result. The former, is reasoning from particulars to the general law; the latter, from effect to cause. The former classifies, the latter explains. [48, p. 194]

In a later series of lectures Peirce expanded and clarified his ideas in the following ways:

> The second figure of reasoning is Retroduction. Here, not only is there no definite probability to the conclusion, but no definite probability attaches even to the mode of inference. We can only say that

the Economy of Research prescribes that we should at a given state of our inquiry try a given hypothesis, and we are to hold to it provisionally as long as the facts will permit. There is no probability about it. It is a mere suggestion which we tentatively adopt. [49, p. 142]

As for retroduction, it is itself an experiment. ... It begins always with colligation, of course, of a variety of separately observed facts about the subject of the hypothesis. ... Something corresponding to iteration may or may not take place. And then comes an Observation. Not, however, an External observation of the objects as in Induction, nor yet an Observation made upon the parts of a Diagram, as in Deduction; but for all that just as truly an observation. ... Now the surrender which we make in Retroduction, is a surrender to the Insistence of an Idea. The hypothesis, as The Frenchman says, *c'est plus fort que moi*. It is irresistible; it is imperative. We must throw open our galis and admit it, at any rate for the time being. [49, p. 170]

The kind of inference Peirce is describing can perhaps best be illustrated by thinking of the final scene in many classical detective novels. All the suspects are gathered in one room, and the detective (Sherlock Holmes, Hercule Poirot, or Miss Marple) walks in, points a finger at the guilty person, and lays out the whole plot. The reasoning leading to this conclusion is abductive, it seeks the explanation that best fits the available data; but after the conclusion has been reached (the guilty one discovered and pointed out), the scene is not over; the detective then uses inductive and deductive reasoning to show that what is postulated is really the best explanation (e.g., 'it could not have been the butler because he was ten miles away at the time of the crime'). In this way, abduction establishes a hypothesis which then has to be tested against the available data, and new data which may be discovered. The inference is therefore only admitted as valid 'for the time being'.

Whether or not abduction is a separate mode of inference from deduction and induction is a question that has vexed philosophers for quite some time. Consider a simple abduction such as: there are footprints on the beach; probably, therefore, a person has walked along the beach recently. Arguments such as this can be reconstructed as either deductive or inductive

[50]. But this does not show that all abductions can be reconstructed in this way. It may be that even abductions explaining a large number of 'observations' can be represented as a
network of deductive and inductive inferences, but there is no
way to prove that this is the case, and it seems at least doubtful if the set of 'observations' contains contradictory elements.
In a recent book Peter Lipton has provided an excellent
account of the problems in inference to the best explanation
[51]. The project I am pursuing here has some connections to
his account, but there are also substantial differences. In
Lipton's exposition, causality and the possibility of causal
explanation play a very important role, whereas in my account
causal explanation (if possible) plays a much smaller role.

At this point we can connect Peirce's account of abduction
to the coherence theory of justification in contemporary epistemology, to provide a full account of a valid analytic logic for
qualitative research – an analytic logic that is able to produce
scientific knowledge. According to coherence theory: 'A belief
B1 is justified to the extent to which it contributes to coherence of the belief-set of which it is a member' [40, p. 127]. Justification is a function of the relationship between a belief and
all the other beliefs in the belief-set in which it occurs, and
there is no further foundation for justification. The coherence
theory thereby rejects the traditional foundationalist idea that
a belief can only be justified if it can be placed in a valid infer-
ential chain originating in some piece of evidence that is certain. Coherence theory is compatible with empiricism, if
'beliefs produced by direct sensory perception have an *a priori*
greater security than other beliefs': such beliefs create greater
coherence in a person's belief-set [52].

If we go back to the picture of the qualitative research
process outlined above, we can treat the set of beliefs generated during the process as a separate belief-set, which includes
the prior theoretical and personal beliefs of the researchers
(their horizon of understanding) and the data, and low-level
explanatory hypotheses generated during the research. From
this belief-set, researchers generate an overarching explanation
by abduction (either through some method, or in a 'flash of

insight'). This abduction is itself a further belief which is added to the belief-set, and it is justified if and only if it adds significantly to the coherence of the belief-set. An abductive hypothesis which can explain, and thereby connect, a large number of previously unconnected beliefs in the belief-set is more justified than one which only explains a few. Lipton describes this aspect of evaluating hypothesis as subjunctive assessment: 'Inference to the Best Explanation also suggest that we assess candidate inferences by asking a subjunctive question: we ask how good the explanation *would* be if it were true' [51, p. 67, emphasis in original].

In some cases we will be able to come up with more than one equally plausible abductive hypothesis. In these cases we will have to choose between the contenders, and other factors than the mere likelihood of each of the hypotheses being true must come into play. Lipton makes a distinction between the likeliness and the loveliness of a theory or hypothesis, and defines loveliness in the following way: 'On the other hand, we may characterize the best explanation as the one which would, if correct, be the most explanatory or provide the most understanding: the 'loveliest' explanation' [51, p. 61]. His example of a really lovely theory is Newtonian mechanics, which, in his interpretation, superseded its predecessors not because it fitted the data available at the time better, but because of its 'lovely' explanatory abilities. If we have two or more equally likely hypotheses, it makes sense to choose the loveliest.

As Peirce has already pointed out, an explanation gained by abduction has to be tested, both by going through the available data (beliefs in the belief-set) to see whether there are any that it does not explain, or any that are directly contradictory to the hypothesis, and by seeking new data. When we have a 'flash of insight', we may well believe that it is a better explanation than it shows itself to be when we try to make it fit the total belief-set generated in the research process. The role of method is therefore to guide the process on two levels: first, to ensure that data are generated which are useful in the generation and testing of abductive hypotheses, and second, to promote rigour in the testing process.

The scientific status of qualitative research revisited

This indicates that we can reconstruct the analytic process in qualitative research as an iterative series of hypothesis generation (abduction), hypothesis testing, and hypothesis revision, or, perhaps better, as an iterative series of theory revisions within a single Lakatosian research programme. Lakatos's own three conditions for labelling a change in theory as progressive indicate that a change in a belief-set is justified according to the coherence theory of justification.

If each step in the process was made explicit, and if each step involved the testing of one simple well-defined hypothesis, we could talk of an iterative series of Popperian falsification attempts, alternating between a context of discovery (abduction) and a context of justification. As described above, this degree of explicitness can seldom be reached in qualitative research. The analysis can follow a logic of conjecture and refutation, but the conjectures are more complex, and the procedures for refutation not necessarily experimental. But by combining abduction with rigorous attention to whether our abductive explanations a) really produce coherence in the present belief-set, and b) are able to explain new data, we can make sure that our development of overarching explanations do represent progressive theory shifts. Most of us probably have the intuition that a theory that can explain new data (that is, a theory with some sort of predictive power) is better than a theory that can only explain the data obtained so far. To show that this intuition is correct turns out to be rather difficult, and is outside the scope of the present book. The interested reader is referred to Peter Lipton, *Inference to the Best Explanation*, chapter 8 [51].

If such an analysis process is carried through, we are justified in claiming scientific status for the final inference to best explanation. Whether others are likely to accept the findings as scientifically valid will then depend to what degree this process can be documented. Here it is important to be able to produce a convincing analysis trail, showing exactly how the result was reached.

On the practical level, this account of the scientific status of qualitative research leads to the following methodological rules of thumb:

1. it is important to keep a record of the development of the data analysis;
2. it is preferable that data collection and analysis are not totally separated, so that emerging explanations/theory can be tested against new data;
3. the aim of the analysis is to give an account explaining as much of the data as possible (that is, to create the largest possible subset of coherent beliefs from the total set of beliefs generated, since it is unlikely that any hypothesis will explain all data, or that the set will not contain contradictory data).

Explanation and interpretation

Until now, I have taken it as unproblematic that qualitative researchers are actually studying real phenomena, and that they are able to interpret their data. But both these claims are contentious.

First, there is a general problem facing sociology, economics, political science, etc. that it is unclear what status the structures they claim to study have. Are these fields of study just an extension of group psychology, or do structures such as 'ideology' or 'national interest' have a status which goes beyond being a mere aggregate of individual psychologies? I will leave that question aside here, first, because it is a problem shared by quantitative and qualitative research in these fields, and second, because there is already an extensive literature on the subject [see 53–6].

The second problem emerges from the nature of the data that are used in most qualitative research. These data (interviews, observations, etc.) are generated in an interplay with other human beings. They come to the researcher with certain meanings already attached, and they have to be interpreted before they can be fully understood. If this interpretation is tainted by some form of ineradicable bias, the whole project can be cut off at the root, because this casts doubt on the status of the basic data.

Early in the history of modern hermeneutics, Dilthey posited an absolute dichotomy between explanation and understanding. Explanation (that is, causal explanation) was the scientific aim of the natural sciences, whereas the human sciences aimed to create understanding [57]. This dichotomy was claimed to be absolute, and to constitute a true demarcation between these two kinds of sciences. The establishment of this dichotomy has, however, had unexpected and negative consequences, because the success of the natural sciences has fostered the attitude that the only true scientific achievement is causal explanation.

There has also been a school of criticism internal to the human sciences which has claimed that understanding cannot be achieved, first, because when we interpret we do so on the basis of our own prejudices, and second, because language (even single words) is inescapably polysemic, and cannot be given any fixed meaning.

I am not going to dwell long on the last objection, which has been most forcefully argued by Derrida [58]. It seems to me to take a small true insight and expand it to absurd proportions. It may well be true that language is polysemic to some extent, but since we are able to communicate quite well in daily life, it cannot be the case that its polysemic nature prevents the local fixation of meaning, because if it did, we could not communicate. And if Derrida's assertions were true, he himself would be in a situation where he could not communicate them to others, because he would have to do so through the ineluctably polysemic structure of language. So the mere fact that Derrida continues to write books (if these books are intended to say something to somebody), should make us wary of his project.

Hermeneutics and prejudice

The first objections — that the only true form of scientific achievement is explanation, and that understanding is blocked by our own prejudices — are more important, and I will try to answer them in the reverse order in which they are stated here.

The aim of early modern hermeneutics was to establish procedural rules for interpretation which would ensure that the interpreter reached a true and unbiased account of the meaning of the text being interpreted. This project floundered early in this century, because no such rules could be produced. There always remained a residual element of personal choice in the interpretative process. Because the humanities and the social sciences are building on data which have to be interpreted, this could vitiate their claim to produce scientific knowledge.

One possible solution to this problem was put forward by Gadamer in his very influential book *Truth and Method* [59]. He argues, that it is true that our understanding and our interpretation are always influenced by our prejudices (Vorurteile), but that this is not necessarily an insurmountable problem for hermeneutics as a scientific discipline. It only becomes a problem if our goal is a method which will, in and of itself, produce knowledge that is guaranteed to be true; and, as we saw above, a falsificationist approach to the philosophy of science acknowledges that science does not produce certain knowledge.

Gadamer takes his point of departure in Heidegger's analysis of the forestructures of perception and understanding. According to this analysis, our perception of the world is always already a function of our preconceptions, prejudices, and presumptions. We do not have direct access to the world as it is, and even less direct access to the meanings expressed by other people. Because this is an inescapable feature of human existence, there is no purpose in perceiving it purely as a negative hindrance to understanding. Gadamer argues that without this forestructure we could not even begin to understand each other. It is only because there is an overlap between my forestructure (or in Gadamer's terms my horizon of understanding) and the forestructure of the other that we can understand each other.

It is also important to note that prejudices are not

unchangeable. Just like the legal term 'prejudication', which is the etymological root of prejudice, a prejudice may be changed in the light of further evidence. The process of interpretation must therefore include a constant questioning of the interpreter's own prejudices.

According to Gadamer, the purpose of a process of interpretation is to achieve a fusion of horizons of understanding, so that each participant gains full insight into the other person's horizon of understanding. This is the ideal outcome, and Gadamer fully realises that it is not achievable, but nevertheless claims that this is the ideal one ought to strive for (that is, it is a regulative ideal for the process).

When the interpreter belongs to the same culture as the producer of the text he is interpreting, he can use the shared tradition and his knowledge of the 'effective history' of words and phrases to help in the interpretative task, because words and utterances only gain meaning through their 'effective history' inscribed in tradition. In this way Gadamer seeks to rehabilitate both prejudice and tradition as important positive factors in interpretation.

Because the fusion of horizons is only a regulative ideal, the hermeneutic process will never lead to a full understanding of the other (that is, it will never lead to the 'truth' about the text in an absolute sense), but it can lead to an understanding which is better – fuller and deeper – than that gained without interpretation, and this is sufficient to lay claim to scientific status, or, in Gadamer's own words:

> Thus there is undoubtedly no understanding that is free of all prejudices, however much the will of our knowledge must be directed towards escaping their thrall. It has emerged throughout our investigation that the certainty that is imparted by the use of scientific methods does not suffice to guarantee truth. This is so especially of the human sciences, but this does not mean a diminution of their scientific quality, but, on the contrary, the justification of the claim to special humane significance that they have always made. The fact that in the knowing involved in them the knower's own being is involved marks, certainly, the limitation of 'method', but not that of science. Rather, what the tool of method does not achieve must

– and effectively can – be achieved by a discipline of questioning and research, a discipline that guarantees truth. [59, p. 447]

Gadamer's rehabilitation of tradition in hermeneutics was criticised in the late 1960s and early 1970s by Habermas and others, who claimed that it neglected the systematically distorting function of ideology [26, 60]. Habermas wants to take this into account, and to return to a 'hermeneutics of suspicion' which distrusts immediate meaning, and traces it back to an unconscious or conscious interest/ideology. This move is already anticipated by Gadamer, who has never just advocated a non-critical and non-reflective acceptance of tradition. Hermeneutics always aims at critically reflexive knowledge, and in this process the authority of any tradition is always tentative.

Ricoeur expands this insight by pointing out that a critique of ideology presupposes an interpretation of ideology, and a true hermeneutics presupposes a distantiation from the self, which allows the text to speak. If such a distantiation can be accomplished, a critique of ideology can become an integral part of the hermeneutic process, and Habermas' critical point of view can be integrated within Gadamer's hermeneutics. What Gadamer has shown is that, although interpretation builds on prejudice, this does not invalidate the process or the outcome.

Explanation and understanding

The objection that the only true form of scientific achievement is causal explanation must also be taken seriously, since its truth would entail that large parts of the humanities and social sciences would not meet the mark. It is often not possible to produce an explanation in a traditional causal form, where the outcome is invariably predicted by a given initial situation and a set of causal laws.

This does not, however, imply that causal explanation is not possible in the humanities and social sciences. In *Explanation and Understanding* von Wright offers the example of the outbreak of the First World War [61]. Can we claim as a valid explanation that the cause of the outbreak of the war was the assassination of the Austrian Archduke at Sarajevo in June 1914? According to von Wright, such a claim is valid, because the *explanans* (the assassination) can be connected to the *explanandum* (the outbreak of the war) through a series of practical syllogisms influencing the main actors in the scenario (the Austrian, Serbian, and Russian governments). These practical syllogisms do not establish a nomic connection between *explanans* and *explanandum*, but they do establish a fully sufficient causal link by taking the motivational background of the main actors into account. Von Wright calls this kind of explanation quasi-causal, not because they are not causal, but because they do not establish nomic connections.

The objection that causal explanations is the only true scientific achievement can also be met in another way by pointing out, that causal explanation is not the only available form of explanation. In the interpretation of texts, structural explanations can be much more important in trying to understand the meaning and message of the text. This point has been argued by Paul Ricoeur, who tries to show that in the discourse with a text explanation precedes understanding [62]. It is only when we have explained the text, either by explaining its structure or the quasi-causal relations underlying the text, that we can truly understand it.

Ricoeur does not accept the structuralist claim, that when the structure of a text has been elucidated the text is fully understood [63]. He claims that the narrative of the text is more than its structure, but he does accept the validity of structural elucidation as an important part in the process of interpretation:

> I shall therefore say: to explain is to bring out the structure, that is, the internal relations of dependence which constitute the statics of the text; to interpret is to follow the path of thought opened up by the text, to place oneself *en route* towards the *orient* of the text. We are invited by this remark to correct our initial concept of interpretation and to search – beyond a subjective process of interpretation as an act *on* the text – for an objective process of interpretation which would be the act *of* the text.' [62, pp. 161–2, emphasis in original]

In this way, the antithetical dichotomy between explanation and understanding is resolved, and both are shown to be important for the development of an interpretation of a text.

Initial interpretation and the basis of analysis

In a qualitative research project of the kind discussed here the initial interpretation of the data collected through interviews or observation is only the first step in a long analytic process. But it is only when we understand each individual piece of datum, that we are able to move on to a comparison and further analysis. The last two sections have endeavoured to show, that although this initial interpretation must necessarily proceed from a certain horizon of understanding, this does not necessarily bias the interpretation in a damaging way. By maintaining a critical attitude, and by employing explanatory methods, the interpretative process can yield an understanding of the data which is fully sufficient to form part of the basis of a claim to scientific status.

Notes

1 A theory stating that truth is, in the final analysis, decided by correspondence between the statement in question and reality. This seems to be the common-sense approach to truth, but requires further elaboration to be philosophically tenable. The standard formalisation is that given by Tarski [11].

2 A theory stating that truth is, in the final analysis, decided by whether or not a given assertion is useful in practical life. The original formulation of this theory is that given by the American pragmatist William James [11]. The leading contemporary pragmatist Richard Rorty has recently suggested that we should discard the concept of truth altogether [12].

3 This follows from the unsymmetrical nature of the two argumentation schemata below where (1) is invalid and (2) is valid:

(1)	(2)
A implies B	A implies B
B	not B
therefore A	therefore not A

References

1 Heidegger, M., *Basic Writings*. San Fransisco: Harper Collins, 1993.

2 Lægeforeningens Forskningspolitiske Udvalg. *Et tilløb til en forskningspolitik*. København: Lægeforeningen, 1995.

3 Jungersen, D., Forpremiere på en forskningspolitik. *Ugeskrift for Læger* 1995; 157: 3501–5.

4 Tschudi, F., Do qualitative and quantitative methods require different approaches to validity? In: Kvale, S. (ed.), *Issues of Validity in Qualitative Research*. Lund: Studentlitteratur, 1989: pp. 109–34.

5 Polkinghorne, D. E., *Methodology for the Human Sciences*. Albany, NY: SUNY Press, 1983.

6 Kvale, S., To validate is to question. In: Kvale, S. (ed.), *Issues of Validity in Qualitative Research*. Lund: Studentlitteratur, 1989: pp. 73–92.

7 Kuhn, T. S., *The Structure of Scientific Revolutions* (2nd edn). Chicago: University of Chicago Press, 1970.

8 Leininger, M., Evaluation criteria and critique of qualitative research studies. In: Morse, J. M., (ed.), *Critical Issues in Qualitative Research Methods*. Thousand Oaks, CA: Sage Publications, 1994: pp. 95-115.

9 Lunde, I. M., *Patienters egenvurdering – et medicinsk perspektivskift*. København: FADL's Forlag, 1990.

10 Launsø, L., Rieper, O., *Forskning om og med mennesker – Metoder og vilkår i samfundsforskning*. København: Nyt Nordisk Forlag, 1987.

11 Tugendhat, E., Wolf, U., *Logisch-semantische Propädeutik*. Stuttgart: Philipp Reclam, jun., 1986.

12 Rorty, R., Is truth a goal of enquiry? Davidson *vs.* Wright. *The Philosophical Quarterly* 1995; 45: 281–300.

13 Salner, M., Validity in human science research. In: Kvale, S. (ed.), *Issues of Validity in Qualitative Research*. Lund: Studentlitteratur, 1989: pp. 47–71.

14 Glover, J. (ed.), *The Philosophy of Mind*. Oxford: Oxford University Press, 1976.

15 Kristensen, K., Madsen, H., Mortensen, P. S,. *Analyse af Kvalitative Data – En Grundbog for Samfundsvidenskaberne* (2nd edn). Herning: Systime, 1986.

16 Miles, M. B., Huberman, A. M., *Qualitative Data Analysis* (2nd edn). Thousand Oaks: Sage Publications, 1994.

17 Ray, M. A., The richness of phenomenology: philosophic, theoretic, and methodological concerns. In: Morse, J. M. (ed.), *Critical Issues in Qualitative Research Methods*. Thousand Oaks, CA: Sage Publications, 1994: pp. 117–33.

18 Cohen, M. Z., Omery, A., Schools of phenomenology: implications for

research. In: Morse, J. M, (ed.), *Critical Issues in Qualitative Research Methods*. Thousand Oaks, CA: Sage Publications, 1994: pp. 136–56.

19 Hammond, M., Howarth, J., Keat, R., *Understanding Phenomenology*. Oxford: Blackwell Publishers, 1991.

20 Kolakowski, L., *Husserl and the Search for Certitude*. Chicago: University of Chicago Press, 1987.

21 Heritage, J., *Garfinkel and Ethnomethodology*. Cambridge: Polity Press, 1962.

22 Schutz, A., *Collected Papers: The Problem of Social Reality*. The Hague: Martinus Nijhoff Publishers, 1962.

23 Gergen, K. J., Gergen, M. M., Toward reflexive methodologies. In: Steier, F. (ed.), *Research and Reflexivity*. London: Sage Publications, 1991.

24 Latour, B., *The Pasteurization of France*. Cambridge, MA: Harvard University Press, 1988.

25 Payer, L., *Medicine and Culture – Notions of Health and Sickness*. London: Victor Gollancz, 1990.

26 Habermas, J., *Toward a Rational Society – Student Protest, Science, and Politics*. Boston: Beacon Press, 1970.

27 Habermas, J., *The Theory of Communicative Action* (vol. 1). Boston: Beacon Press, 1984.

28 Habermas, J., *The Theory of Communicative Action* (vol. 2). Boston: Beacon Press, 1987.

29 Wagner, L., *Innovation in Primary Health Care for Elderly People in Denmark – Two Action Research Projects*. Gothenburg: The Nordic School of Public Health, 1994.

30 Dunn, J., Urmson, J. O., Hume, A. J., *The British Empiricists: Locke, Berkeley, Hume*. Oxford: Oxford University Press, 1992.

31 Feyerabend, P., *Against Method* (3rd edn). London: Verso, 1993.

32 Popper, K. R., *The Logic of Scientific Discovery*. New York: Basic Books, 1959 (org. Logik der Forschung, 1934).

33 Moody, L. E., *Advancing Nursing Science Through Research* (vol. 1). Newbury Park, CA: Sage Publications, 1990.

34 Losee, J., *A Historical Introduction to the Philosophy of Science* (3rd edn). Oxford: Oxford University Press, 1993.

35 Popper, K. R., *Objective Knowledge: An Evolutionary Approach*. Oxford: Oxford University Press, 1972.

36 Quine, W. V. O., *From a Logical Point of View*. Cambridge, MA: Harvard University Press, 1953.

37 Lakatos, I., Falsification and the methodology of scientific research programs. In: Lakatos, I., Musgrave, A. (eds), *Criticism and the Growth of*

Knowledge. Cambridge: Cambridge University Press, 1970: pp. 91–196.

38 Chalmers, A. F., *What is this thing called Science?* (2nd edn). Buckingham: Open University Press, 1982.

39 Plato, *Theaetetus*. 201c–202d. One translation can be found in: Cornford, F. M. (tran.), *Plato's Theory of Knowledge – The Theaetetus and the Sophist of Plato*. New York: Macmillan Publishing Company, 1957.

40 Dancy, J., *Introduction to Contemporary Epistemology*. Oxford: Blackwell Publishers, 1985.

41 Gettier, E. L., Is justified true belief knowledge? *Analysis*, 1963; 23: 121–3.

42 Moser, P. K., Gettier problem. In: Dancy, J., Sosa, E. (eds), *A Companion to Epistemology*. Oxford: Blackwell Publishers, 1993: pp. 157–9.

43 Strauss, A., Corbin, J., *Basics of Qualitative Research – Grounded Theory Procedures and Techniques*. Newbury Park, CA: Sage Publications, 1990.

44 Robrecht, L. C., Grounded theory: evolving methods. *Qualitative Health Research* 1995; 5: 169–77.

45 Munhall, P. L., Qualitative designs. In: Brink, P. J., Wood, M. J., *Advanced Design in Nursing Research*. Newbury Park, CA: Sage Publications, 1989: pp. 161–79.

46 Addison, R. B., Grounded hermeneutic research. In: Crabtree, B. F., Miller, W. L. (eds), *Doing Qualitative Research*. Newbury Park, CA: Sage Publications, 1992: pp. 110–24.

47 Corrington, R. S., *An Introduction to C. S. Peirce – Philosopher, Semiotician, and Ecstatic Naturalist*. Lanham, MD: Rowman and Littlefield Publishers, 1993.

48 Peirce, C. S., Deduction, induction, and hypothesis (1878). In: Houser, N., Kloesel C. (eds), *The Essential Peirce – Selected Philosophical Writings* (vol. 1). Bloomington: Indiana University Press, 1992: pp. 186–99.

49 Peirce, C. S., Reasoning and the logic of things (1898). In: Ketner, K.L. (ed.), *Reasoning and the Logic of Things – Charles Sanders Peirce*. Cambridge, MA: Harvard University Press, 1992.

50 Fumerton, R., Inference to the best explanation. In: Dancy, J., Sosa, E. (eds), *A Companion to Epistemology*. Oxford: Blackwell Publishers, 1993: pp. 207–9.

51 Lipton, P., *Inference to the Best Explanation*. London: Routledge, 1991.

52 Dancy, J. P., On coherence theories of justification: can an empiricist be a coherentist? *American Philosophical Quarterly* 1984; 21: 359–65.

53 Hughes, J., *The Philosophy of Social Research* (2nd edn). London: Longman, 1990.

54 Hollis, M., *The Philosophy of Social Science – An Introduction*. Cambridge: Cambridge University Press, 1994.

55 Boyd, R., Gasper, P., Trout, J. D. (ed.), *The Philosophy of Science*. Cam-

bridge, MA: MIT Press, 1991.

56 Craib, I., *Modern Social Theory – From Parsons to Habermas*. Brighton: Wheatsheaf Books, 1984.

57 Grondin, J., *Introduction to Philosophical Hermeneutics*. New Haven: Yale University Press, 1994.

58 Derrida, J., *Writing and Difference*. London: Routledge and Kegan Paul, 1978.

59 Gadamer, H-G., *Truth and Method*. London: Sheed and Ward Ltd., 1975.

60 Ricoeur P., Hermeneutics and the critique of ideology. In: Thompson, J. B. (ed.), *Paul Ricoeur – Hermeneutics and the Human Sciences*. Cambridge: Cambridge University Press, 1981: pp. 63–100.

61 von Wright, G. H., *Explanation and Understanding*. Ithaca, NY: Cornell University Press, 1971.

62 Ricoeur, P., What is a text? Explanation and understanding. In: Thompson, J. B. (ed.), *Paul Ricoeur – Hermeneutics and the Human Sciences*. Cambridge: Cambridge University Press, 1981: pp. 145–164.

63 Sturrock, J., *Structuralism*. London: Paladin Grafton Books, 1986.

4

Protective responsibility: a core notion in the ethical reasoning of health care professionals

There was no room left for casuistry. To weigh one passion against the other, with the discordant voices of honour and expedience dinning in his ears, had too long involved him in fruitless torture. Both were right: neither could be surrendered. If the facts showed them irreconcilable, *tant pis pour les faits*. A way must be found to satisfy both or neither. [1, p. 179]

We would like to know what, as moral agents, we have got to do because of logic, what we have got to do because of human nature, and what we can choose to do. [2, p. 2]

Studying moral reasoning

The subject of this book is the moral reasoning of doctors and nurses. After three chapters of introduction, philosophical argument for the importance of empirical ethics and for the scientific status of qualitative research, I am now finally able to move on to the actual empirical study. This chapter will first present a brief account of the reasons for choosing the methodology used in the study, and then move on to the main results and present a description of how health care professionals identify ethical problems, and how they reason about the problems they have identified.

Choosing methodology

A basic problem in all research on ethical reasoning is the choice of research methodology. Data can be collected in a variety of ways, and may be analysed with a variety of different methods (see Table 4.1). Each of these methods has its own strengths and weaknesses, and the choice of methodology will in the end be determined by a balancing of these factors, and by what is practically possible.

Table 4.1   Choices of methodology

Data collection:	Analysis:
questionnaires	quantitative
standardised	semi-quantitative
ad hoc	content analysis
interviews	qualitative
structured	hermeneutics
semi-structured	classical
unstructured	new
focus groups	critical
participant observation	phenomenology
covert observation	grounded theory
experimental approaches	

Data collection

There is no doubt that covert observation is a very strong method for gathering data on the actual ethical-decision-making by health care professionals. But covert observation also creates so many ethical problems about the consent of the persons involved, and about the way in which such data can be published, that the method must be rejected in all cases where the subject of the research is in any way sensitive (and this is definitely the case with ethical decision-making) [3]. The problem of consent concerns both those who are the direct objects of the study (that is, in this case, health care personnel), and those who incidentally become research objects because they interact with the primary objects of study (that is, patients). This means that it is not sufficient to obtain the consent of health care personnel (and carry out participant observation); the consent of the patients would also have to be secured. In several recent Danish observation projects in nursing science, there have, as far as can be ascertained from the published reports, been no attempts to gain consent from the patients [4–6], but I have no wish to emulate this ethically questionable approach. It would, indeed, be strange to study ethical reasoning by unethical methods, although, of course, many social scientists are very permissive in their view of covert research [7–10].

Participant observation is probably the second best method for studying ethical decision-making, but may not, as with covert observation, generate sufficient data for a study of the reasoning behind the decisions, unless these reasons are stated in a public forum as part of the decision-making process, since we can very seldom justifiably infer thought from action (the intentionalist fallacy). The initial plan for this work did contain an observation study of an official body, in which a large part of the discussion time was concerned with ethical issues. This particular study could not, however, be carried out because of problems in securing access.

Focus groups are also a possibility [11, 12], but there are no extant studies using this approach to study ethical reasoning. The method could probably be modified to such studies, but this would be a major task and outside the possibilities of a project focusing on the content of ethical reasoning, and not exclusively on methodology.

Experimental approaches require a prior knowledge of the factors to be varied between the different experimental groups, and require the possibility to influence these factors. Both requirements are difficult to fulfil in a study of ethical reasoning. Unless one accepts a priori a specific theoretical account of ethical reasoning, or at most two or three to be compared, there is no way to define the relevant factors to be studied. I have argued in Chapter 1 that both the main contenders for a psychological theory of moral development and reasoning are deficient, and this in itself precludes the most obvious

experimental designs where these two theories would be compared. Finally, experimental designs are most suitable when
the research question is of the form 'what influences/deter-
mines X?', and not so suitable when the question is of the form
'what is the content of X?'. An experimental design would thus
be optimal in a study of the influence of organisational features on ethical reasoning, but less suitable in a study of the
form and content of ethical reasoning.

Questionnaires share the problem of prior theoretical decisions with experimental studies. Standardised questionnaires
explicitly build on some theoretical framework, but even *ad
hoc* questionnaires have to be based on some specific prior conception of the relevant questions, and the room for new and
really surprising answers will always be limited. Because the
present study was intended to be exploratory and as open as
possible, it was decided not to use questionnaires.

Because of the problems outlined above I decided to use
interviews as the main method of data collection, although
they, too, have their share of methodological problems. There
is the problem of 'conformist respondents' answering in the
way they perceive as socially desirable, and the interaction
between interviewer and respondent may also create an
unwanted bias (the so-called 'interviewer effect') [13]. One
way to try to minimise these effects is by using a fully structured questionnaire, but this again requires a prior choice of
theoretical framework, and it generates a situation which is
often closer to an interrogation than to an interview (or to a
conversation).

The other end of the spectrum is the totally unstructured
interview, where the researcher does not have any checklist or
interview guide, but just tries to engage the respondent in an
open dialogue about the research subject. In its ideal form the
unstructured interview is a fiction. The researcher cannot
avoid having some form of mental checklist of areas that must
be covered in the dialogue. The absence of a written interview
guide or checklist also creates an important methodological
problem, because it makes it more difficult to ensure that all
important areas are covered in every interview [14]. Because

of this, the knowledge of the respondents is not maximally utilised, and the research process becomes less efficient.

I therefore chose to have a written checklist containing the areas to be covered in the interview as well as model questions within each area. In addition, I included case-studies with possible ethical problems in order to develop more data on how such problems were identified by the respondents, how they were distinguished from other problems, and how different ethical considerations were balanced. The interviewguide contained questions pertaining to all steps of the working model of ethical decision-making shown in Figure 4.1, which was influenced by the model of ethical decision-making put forward by James Rest [15, 16].

Figure 4.1 Working model of ethical decision-making

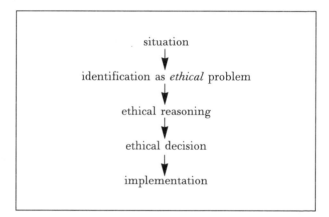

situation

identification as *ethical* problem

ethical reasoning

ethical decision

implementation

Analysis methods

In any kind of research it is important to choose the analysis method and the data collection method at the same time [17]. It is also important that the method fits the questions asked, and not the other way around. In the present study the choice of analysis method was complicated by the subject-matter of the study (ethical reasoning). Moral philosophy has a history that goes back more than 2,500 years, during which time many normative theories have been proposed which describe how persons ought to reason about ethical problems [18]. An important decision was, therefore, what influence theories of moral philosophy (philosophical ethics) should be given in the construction of the interview guide and in the analysis phase.

Professional codes of ethics as basis for analysis

Because the focus is on doctors and nurses, their professional codes of ethics could also play a role in the analysis phase. One of the instruments that have been used in a number of studies of ethical decision-making in nursing is Ketefian's Judgments about Nursing Decisions (JAND) scale, which is constructed to measure conformity with the American Nurses Association (ANA) code of ethics [19]. Some research has found that performance on this scale is positively correlated with levels of nursing education, and moral reasoning measured by Rest's DIT-scale [19], although other researchers have been unable to replicate these findings [20].

The present data could have been analysed by taking the development of the JAND scale as a paradigm example. This would entail identifying the equivalent of 'professionally valued and ideal nursing behaviors that are congruent with the principles expressed in the *Code for Nurses*' [19, p. 13] in the ethical codes of Danish doctors and nurses, and applying the identified categories in an analysis of the interviews. There are at least three reasons why a reliance on professional codes in the analysis of ethical decision-making is problematic.

First, there is no justification for believing that all the prescriptions in professional codes exemplify ideal ethical values. Second, there is evidence that the prescriptions play only a very limited role in the ethical reasoning of professionals. In an American study Cox found that only 6.9 per cent of nurses report using the ANA code as the basis of their ethical decision-making [21]. In Northern Europe professional codes of ethics have even less status than in the USA, so it is likely that their influence is even smaller. This was also found to be the case in the present study. There are very few references to professional codes, and, furthermore, some of these quote the codes wrongly.

Finally, the ethical codes of Danish doctors and nurses, which should have been the basis of such an analysis, are fairly short and non-specific. The current ethical code of the Danish Medical Association, adopted in 1989, contains nineteen very general paragraphs; only the three on information, confidentiality, and biomedical research have specific advice relevant to the ethical problems that occur in clinical work [22]. An analysis based on this code would therefore be extremely narrow.

For these reasons no analytic categories were derived from the professional codes.

The choice of grounded theory

I chose grounded theory as the main analysis method for this study for two reasons: there is an extensive and fairly clear methodological literature [23–8], and the method is compatible with standard assumptions in the philosophy of science.

Grounded theory methodology prescribes a structured approach to data analysis with clearly defined steps, and I will freely admit that this feature appealed to the more quantitative side of my scientific *persona*. But, apart from this, the structured nature of the methodology, and its emphasis on the actual spoken statements of the respondents, make it very suitable for studying ethical reasoning, which as a subject lies at the interface of psychology, sociology, decision-making theory, and moral philosophy. With grounded theory methodology it is possible to focus not only on the psychology, but also on those sociological factors that influence ethical reasoning.

The only other analytic methodology that was seriously considered before the initiation of the study was the phenomenological approach developed by Giorgi [29, 30]. I decided not to use this method, mainly because there is only a tenuous connection between it and its supposed basis in philosophical phenomenology.

Ethical dilemma or ethical problem

The first methodological decision in which moral theory

played a role concerned the terminology used in the interview. Should respondents be asked about 'ethical/moral dilemmas' or about 'ethical/moral problems'? In common parlance there is probably no great difference between the two. For the moral philosopher, however, ethical dilemma has a precise technical meaning, which distinguishes it from ethical problems. For the philosopher, an ethical dilemma occurs when, after full consideration of all relevant factors, I find myself in a situation in which I ought to do two different and mutually exclusive acts. That is, I ought to do act A and at the same time I ought to do act B, but I cannot do both. I am therefore in a situation in which I cannot fulfil all my moral obligations.

Many moral philosophers do not believe that moral dilemmas in this sense exist, which is an important consideration against using this concept as one of the central categories in an analysis of moral thinking. Most consequentialists/utilitarians would, for instance, reject the existence of moral dilemmas. If the utility is the same for both actions, you can just toss a coin, and the action you choose will then be the right one, and there will be no reason to feel regret for not being able to perform both actions. All true Kantians would also reject ethical dilemmas, but for different reasons.

A moral problem has a broader connotation, and does not necessarily imply that the problem is irresolvable. It is possible to be in a situation where it is initially uncertain what act one ought, morally speaking, to perform, but where this uncertainty is dispelled on further deliberation. If for instance, I consider how much of the truth about a serious medical condition I ought to tell a patient who seems to be psychologically fragile, I may have an ethical problem, but I do not necessarily have an ethical dilemma. Furthermore, one study has shown that health care professionals do not identify morally problematic situations as dilemmas, when directly asked. The Nursing Dilemma Test developed by Crisham contains descriptions of six morally problematic situations derived from extensive interviews with nurses. As the name of the test indicates, Crisham has chosen situations which she and her respondents see as dilemmas [31]. In a subsequent study Keller took the same six situations and asked her respondents 'Was it a dilemma for you?' She found that on average they only identified 2.691 of them as dilemmas [32] – that is, less than half of the situations which were presumably dilemmas were identified as such. These results indicate that 'ethical dilemma' may be a somewhat fuzzy concept in common usage.

This conclusion is further supported by a Canadian study which shows that nurses define ethical dilemmas in four different ways; a) as conflicts between the nurse's own principles and those of other professionals, b) as confusion when no obvious right or wrong choice existed, c) as situations where someone's conduct was considered emotionally instead of rationally based, or d) as defined by specific dilemma situations (e.g., concerning the termination of treatment situations) [33]

Given the theoretical disagreement on the very existence of ethical dilemmas, and the practical problems in using the concept consistently, it seemed safer to use the less ambitious concept of ethical problem in the interviews and analysis. And it was decided to use the following broad definition: a person faces an ethical problem in a situation in which ethical considerations are important for the choice of action.

This definition contains many concepts that are philosophically interesting, in the sense that there is no general agreement about their meaning ('person', 'ethical considerations', 'choice', 'action'). For the present purposes it is, fortunately, only necessary to clarify one of these concepts, namely 'ethical considerations'. The other concepts appear in the definition with their common-sense meaning, and no technical specification is necessary here.

Ethical considerations could mean many things, and one of the tasks of metaethics and normative ethics is to clarify the exact meaning of this term and its precise extension. This entails that the concept will have a different meaning and content in different normative theories. A consequentialist and a deontologist will not agree about which considerations are really ethical considerations, and which are not. Since the present study is descriptive, the definition of ethical consideration used here has to be able to encompass both the consequentialist and the deontological considerations, as well as all other considerations that will be called ethical or moral by non-philosophers. In this study, a consideration is therefore classified as an ethical consideration if it: a) refers to a non-legal or not solely legal norm, duty, obligation or right; or b) refers to consequences (well-being, happiness etc.) for some specifiable person or groups of persons; or c) refers to what kind of person one ought to be or what virtues one ought to have.

Moral theory and the analysis of ethical reasoning

The analysis of the data on ethical reasoning could have proceeded exclusively within one of the classical theories of ethics or within one of the more recent frameworks proposed for bioethics. It would, for instance, have been possible to perform an analysis from the perspective of Kantian deontology, consequentialism, virtue ethics, natural law theory, or the more recent four principles approach to bioethics suggested by Beauchamp and Childress and popularised in Europe by Gillon [34–6].

Modern bioethical theory

I have elsewhere analysed modern American bioethics in general, and the four principles approach in particular [37, 38]. I argue that the American approaches are not sufficient as the basis for a normative bioethics, and that, furthermore, they are not suitable as a basis for analysis in empirical studies in ethics.

An analysis of the four principles put forward by Beauchamp and Childress (respect for autonomy, non-maleficence, beneficence, justice) shows that they are clearly influenced by the American context from which they are derived. Autonomy becomes the paramount consideration, and beneficence and justice are neglected. To be useful in Europe, the content of the principles must be redefined. There is also reason to believe that, even if all four principles were given more content, there would still be important areas of the ethical field that would not be covered.

The data collected here could, in principle, be analysed

within the four principles approach, but it would require the development of a new theoretical content of the four principles to accomplish the transfer from an American to a European context. Because of the theoretical worries that I have outlined [37, 38], and the practical problems in the transfer from an American to a European context, I decided not to let the four principles approach influence the analysis presented here.

Another modern approach to medical ethics which could have been used as the basis of the analysis is the 'ethical grid' of the British philosopher David Seedhouse. Seedhouse proposed this grid in 1988 as a tool for moral reasoning in health care [39], but it could possibly also be used as an analytical tool aiding the categorisation of moral statements. The grid has four central ethical values: create autonomy, respect autonomy, serve needs before wants, and respect persons equally. These central values are then surrounced by three further layers of other moral considerations. According to Seedhouse, the inner layer of the grid is concerned with the considerations which form the deep rationale of the model, the next two layers correspond with deontological and consequentialist theory, and the outer layer constitutes the level of external considerations.

The grid builds on Seedhouse's concept of health, and his insistence that the proper role of health care is to work to enhance health. He defines health in the following way:

> A person's optimum state of health is equivalent to the state of the set of conditions which fulfil or enable a person to work to fulfil his or her realistic chosen and biological potentials. Some of these conditions are of the highest importance for all people. Others are variable dependent upon individual abilities and circumstances. [40, p. 61]

Seedhouse's concept of health is partially congruent with our ordinary notions of health and healthiness, but at the same time it includes much more. Although not as broad as the much maligned World Health Organisation (WHO) definition (complete physical, social, and mental well-being), it is still very broad, and it makes it almost impossible to establish a useful demarcation between what is 'work for health' on the one side, and what is 'work for the general benefit of human-ity' on the other. The special moral status that Seedhouse wants to give to work for health therefore becomes doubtful.

Can the grid be used as a method for analysis of empirical data on ethical reasoning? If it is conceptualised solely as a system of categories useful in classifying ethical statements, it can probably be separated from Seedhouse's concept of health, and the arguments against that concept will then not affect the usefulness of the grid. There are, however, other worries about using the grid as the sole classifying scheme.

First, it seems that there are areas of moral life that are left out. There may be many problems with an ethic of care (as pointed out in Chapter 1), but there can be little doubt that it points to an important area of ethical considerations. Like-wise, justice considerations are not unimportant, and they are not fully captured by Seedhouse's 'respect persons equally' con-sideration.

Second the analysis would run into problems at the point where individual statement categories should be put together in some greater whole. Seedhouse does not specify any clear rules describing how to move around in the grid and connect individual categories. There is, therefore, a risk that although statements can be categorised with the grid, the categories remain analytically inert. The framework in which they occur does not contain sufficient resources to link them together, and because the categories are not generated directly from the data they may actually hide connections which are present in the data, but not in the grid.

Based on these considerations I decided not to use the eth-ical grid in the analysis of the data.

Traditional moral philosophy

The two main schools of thought in traditional moral philos-ophy are deontological ethics and consequentialist ethics. The first of these is often connected with Kantian philosophy, whereas the second is generally identified with the utilitarian tradition of Bentham and Mill. But both schools of thought are far wider than these common connections: many deontologists are not Kantians, and some consequentialists are not utilitarians. The best way to distinguish the two schools is probably by focusing on their view of the relation between the right and the good. Deontological ethics defines the right as independent of the good (that is, whether a given act is right does not (only) depends on its consequences). A consequentialist ethics defines the right in terms of the good (that is, whether a given act is right depends only on its consequences) [41, 42].

Aristotle's moral philosophy belongs to neither of these schools, but is based on a concept of virtue (*areté*). The morally good man tries to attain those virtues that are suitable to his position in society, and applies them through proper practical reasoning (*phronesis*). What matters is therefore not the singular act, but that the agent has the right disposition with regard to action. This idea has been revived in recent years, primarily by British philosophers [43], and virtue ethics is today a viable third approach to normative ethics, although there is (not surprisingly) great disagreement regarding the set of characteristics which constitute the proper virtues. The definition of virtue is also contested, but as a working definition MacIntyre's preliminary definition in *After Virtue* seems appropriate, and not too far from the mainstream: 'A virtue is an acquired human quality the possession and exercise of which tends to enable us to achieve those goods which are internal to practices and the lack of which effectively prevents us from achieving any such goods' [44, p. 191].

Another recently resurrected school of moral philosophy is Thomist natural law theory, which has gained adherents both among legal and moral philosophers. The normative structure of this theory resembles a deontological theory fairly closely, but the reasoning behind the normative injunctions builds on an idea about a natural order present in the world and an obligation to follow this order. Traditional natural law theory was developed within the framework of Catholic moral theology, and given its canonical formulation by St Thomas Aquinas [45]. Modern natural law theory is also mainly a school of thought attracting scholars with a Catholic background [46, 47].

The areas covered in the interview guide gave the respondents the opportunity to talk about their own ethical problems, considerations, and reflections, but they were not asked any direct questions aimed at discovering their basic moral theory. The main reason for not doing so is that anyone asked a question such as 'Do you think that the consequences of an act are important when you want to decide whether the act is ethically good or not?' will answer 'Yes', as they will to the question 'Is it wrong to lie to patients?', or to the even more direct question 'Do you have a duty to answer truthfully when patients ask?' It is therefore unlikely that direct questions will be of much help in elucidating the moral theory of non-philosophers. Longer series of 'funnel' questions that gradually target the moral theory of the respondent could be a possibility, but they require a prior specification of the content of the possible theories (otherwise the questions cannot be constructed). This strategy also involves the risk that the respondent is led to a theory through the questions, instead of the questions uncovering the respondent's own theory.

An example of the risk entailed in using very specific questions can be found in the work of Ruess, who wanted to compare the ethical reasoning of health care professionals and parents of infants [48]. Her theoretical framework was the moral theory of Grisez and Boyle (a version of natural law ethics), which divides the moral realm into human goods and principles [49]. Based on this theory, Ruess developed an interview guide in which she directly asked the respondents questions such as 'What values are important in human life?' and 'Did you use the principle of fairness, or the Golden Rule?' [48, p. 108]. Not surprisingly, she found that considerations about human goods and moral principles such as fairness played a substantial role in the moral reasoning of her respondents.

The case-studies presented here were prepared in an attempt to get at least some structured information about the respondents' balancing of different ethical theories and considerations, without having too many leading questions. Some of these cases were specifically constructed to present a problem that could give rise to a conflict between obligations/duties and consequences. No attempt was made to introduce elements in the interview guide explicitly aimed at uncovering traces of virtue ethics or natural law theory.

In the analysis phase it quickly became evident that the ethical reasoning of the respondents was complex, and that an analysis solely in terms of theories from moral philosophy would have to discount large parts of the data. I therefore decided to make two analyses of the data on ethical reasoning: a preliminary analysis looking only at consequentialist and deontological arguments/statements, and a final grounded theory analysis taking into account the totality of the material.

The study

In the following sections I will outline the concrete design decisions which emerged from the methodological considerations mentioned above concerning the interview guide, sampling, and analysis.

The interview guide

The interview guide was constructed with two parts. The first part contained questions about:

1. the last ethical problem the respondents had experienced in their clinical practice;
2. their conception of what it is that makes a problem an ethical problem;
3. their ideas about how ethical problems should be solved;
4. their ideas about the influence patients and family ought to have in the resolution of ethical problems;
5. the influence of the hierarchical structure and other organisational features on the creation, discussion, and solution of ethical problems.

This first part was used as a thematic guide, ensuring that all the areas described were covered, but respondents were not forced to follow one specific route if they themselves moved to a theme 'further down' in the interview guide.

Table 4.2   Short description of case-studies presented

Case number	Description
1.	Clinical trial with drug having side-effects
2.	Clinical trial requiring multiple arterial blood samples
3.	A trial where a pharmaceutical company wants to make yet another in a long row of comparisons of two non-steroid anti-inflamatory drugs (NSAID)
4.	Test of marker for alcoholism. Can blood samples be taken without consent?
5.	Colleague has made error and harmed patient
6.	Elderly patient with prostatic cancer and bronchitis; discussion of 'do-not-resuscitate' order
7.	Elderly patient with congestive heart failure and pneumonia; family states that 'they wish that no theraputic measures should be taken if an exacerbation occurs'
8.	Two patients with cardiac arrest arrive simultaneously in the emergency room
9.	Patient released from hospital after orchiectomy without being told that the histology shows cancer
10.	Elderly patient admitted with pneumonia is restless and agitated at night. Can he be given a sedative against his will?
11.	Operation of HIV-positive patient
12.	Patient with visual acuity below the limit to keep a driving licence
13.	Schizophrenic out-patient refusing to take her medicine

The second half of the interview guide consisted of thirteen case-studies, each presenting a clinical situation containing one or more potential ethical problems (see Table 4.2). The case-studies were selected to represent a range of problems in clinical and research practice, and were discussed extensively with a number of doctors and nurses in clinical work before they were included. For each case the respondents were asked four questions:

1. are there one or more ethical problems in this case?
2. if so, what is the problem(s)?
3. how would you resolve the problem(s), and what ethical considerations would you apply?
4. are there any non-ethical considerations that would influence your decision?

The interview-guide was developed after a study of the relevant literature. A main consideration in the development was to ensure that the first part of the interview was relatively free of any 'interviewer effect', which was why the first question was 'Please tell me about the last ethical problem you experienced in your work?', thereby giving the respondents a chance to use their own words and concepts. The proposed interview-guide was discussed with colleagues, and tested in pilot interviews.

Interview and transcription

The interviews took place in the offices or homes of the respondents and lasted between forty-five minutes and two hours. The interviews were taped, and later transcribed verbatim. All transcriptions were carried out by the same secretary following a detailed guide, and were later verified and corrected by the researcher against the original tape recordings. No attempt was made to capture differences in mood or intonation in the transcription, nor were any explicit contextual markers used.

A transcription with these limitations will inevitably lead to some loss of meaning in the material transcribed, but it was judged in the present context this would be small and that it would be outweighed by the advantages in ease of transcription [50].

Selection of respondents

The study used strategic sampling. The physicians contacted were selected semi-randomly based on the idea that medical specialty, position in the hierarchy, and gender might be connected to differences in ethical outlook. The sampling was therefore designed to maximise the spread of the sample with regard to these characteristics [51].

There are at present more than twenty recognised medical specialties in Denmark, but in order to reduce the number of interviews it was decided only to recruit respondents from ten of these:

1. internal medicine with subspecialties;
2. oncology;
3. paediatrics;
4. geriatrics;
5. orthopaedic surgery;
6. general surgery with subspecialties;
7. gynaecology and obstetrics;
8. anaesthesiology and intensive-care medicine;
9. psychiatry;
10. general practice.

A list was prepared of all hospital departments in these specialties on the island of Sjælland (the main island of Denmark), and a random choice was made of one department in each specialty (two in the case of internal medicine). One consultant was then chosen randomly from each of these departments, and was sent a letter containing a full description of the study and the interview process. About a week later they were contacted by telephone and asked whether they were willing to participate.

After the interviews with the consultants, the department's list of junior medical staff was obtained. A similar process was applied to this list in order to choose one senior registrar and one house officer or registrar from each department. If the person chosen had moved, or could not be contacted by phone within one month of the mailing of the letter, a new person was chosen from the same group.

General practitioners were initially chosen at random from the membership list of the Danish Medical Association, but because of recruitment problems, a convenience sample was eventually used, taken at a meeting for general practitioners in Copenhagen County. A convenience sample of nurses was assembled through a contact in the nursing administration at Frederiksberg Hospital.

In all, thirty-three doctors and nine nurses were recruited, before saturation was reached (that is the phenomenon that after a certain number of interviews no new data are produced, everything said has been heard before). No specific rationale for the selection of this number of respondents can be produced, and the numbers recommended in the methodological literature vary widely from not more than eight [52], to considerably higher numbers [53]. A recent review of sampling in qualitative inquiry states that: 'experience has shown that 6–8 data sources or sampling units will often suffice for a homogeneous sample, while 12–20 commonly are needed when looking for disconfirming evidence or trying to achieve maximum variation' [54, p. 41]. This would indicate that the forty-two people interviewed here constitute an adequate sample for most qualitative purposes. The basic demographic data of the respondents can be found in Table 4.3.

Table 4.3   Demography of respondents

	Doctors		*Nurses*
Sex			
M	25		1
F	8		8
Age range	31–60		26–62
Position			
consultant	11	chief nurse	2
senior registrar	9	assistant chief nurse	2
registrar/house officer	6	staff nurse	5
general practitioner	7		

Analysis

The technical part of the coding process was managed using the computer programs TextBase Alpha for PC and The Etno-

graph v4.0 [55]. TextBase Alpha was initially chosen because
its functions are suitable for grounded theory analysis, and
because it supports most of the functions mentioned in the literature on the use of computers in qualitative research [56].
The functions in The Etnograph are much more advanced, and
the more advanced retrieval functions were especially useful in
later stages of the analysis.

The grounded theory analysis followed the framework
described in Strauss's and Corbin's *Basics of Qualitative
Research* with the modifications necessary for a primarily
descriptive study instead of a theory generating study [23,
26–8]. Previous books by Glaser and Strauss were also studied
prior to the analysis and used as background material [24, 25],
but the direct methodological advice in these earlier works is
not as clearly stated as in the Strauss and Corbin book.

The recent discussion initiated by Glaser about whether
the Strauss and Corbin methodology is a perversion of the original ideas behind the grounded theory approach [57] caused no
changes in the analysis strategy for the present study. Glaser's
main concern is with grounded theory as a theory-generating
methodology, and he sees the Strauss and Corbin approach as
a departure from the theory-generating side of grounded
theory towards what he calls 'full conceptual description' –
that is, description without developing theory. When one com-
pares Strauss's and Corbin's 1990 work [26] with the original
Glaser and Strauss book of 1967 [24], it does seem that Glaser
has a point [58, 59]. It is, however, a point that is of lesser
interest in connection with the present study because the main
aim of this study is in-depth description.

Line by line analysis and open coding was initially performed on a sample of eighteen interviews using the method
of constant comparative analysis. The theoretical and *in vivo*
codes generated by this process were reviewed, certain codes
were discarded as redundant, and the remaining codes were
provisionally arranged under a number of category headings,
and dimensionalised. The coding scheme developed was then
applied to all forty-two interviews. A presumptive core category labelled 'protective responsibility' emerged from this

analysis process, and its validity and relation to other coding categories were elucidated through selective and process coding. Throughout the analytic process memos were written and diagrams and displays used for further clarification [60].

A recent paper in a collection on qualitative methodology mentions the need to have an academic pedigree traceable to either Glaser or Strauss through a series of mentoring relationships in order to perform grounded theory analysis [59]. The present author must admit that he has no such pedigree, and can lay no claim to the blessings of the apostolic succession. It seems, however, that there is an inherent incoherence between the two claims: grounded theory is a scientific methodology, and grounded theory methodology can only be learned in a mentoring relationship.

If grounded theory methodology can only be learned in a mentoring relationship, it must imply that it cannot be learned or understood by studying any public description of the methodology, because otherwise the mentor would not be necessary. But if it cannot be learned or understood from publicly available descriptions, methodology of grounded theory studies cannot be criticised by any who have not themselves learned it through a mentoring relationship, because understanding a methodology is a necessary prerequisite for criticising it or its use. Grounded theory studies would therefore not be open to real external criticism, not even from researchers from closely related fields who have made a thorough study of the available methodological literature. But this in turn puts the claim that grounded theory is a scientific methodology in question. Are we really prepared to call something a *scientific* methodology if it is not open to external criticism? I suspect not, and since the claim to scientific status seems more valuable than the mentoring claim, I will argue that it is the mentoring claim that should be abandoned. This does not suggest that mentoring is not important, but only that mentoring with the correct pedigree cannot be a necessary condition for performing grounded theory studies.

In addition to the grounded theory analysis, longer passages containing ethical argument and discussion were analysed statement for statement, in an attempt to identify the factual and ethical premises used and the conclusions drawn. Individual statements were initially categorised either as right/obligation/duty statements or as consequentialist statements, in an attempt to follow the classical distinction between deontological and teleological theories in moral philosophy. This categorisation was, however, found to be deficient in the sense that it could not be made exhaustive and exclusive unless a significant number of statements were not taken at face value. Two further substantial categories were therefore established, one containing statements concerned with the necessity to build or maintain a good relationship with the patient, and one containing statements about the respect owed to patients as human beings.

The analysis of real life arguments is complicated by two main factors; first, such arguments are often highly enthymematic (that is, they contain many hidden premises), and second, they often use aberrant logics that transgress the rules of first order predicate logic or the prohibitions against circular arguments, but which nevertheless seem to make sense in everyday speech [61–4]. This lack of logic in everyday speech is further supported by a large empirical study of reasoning skills, defined as the ability to reason without manifest or implicit inconsistency, which has shown that very few people are actually able to perform this task consistently, and that subject experts are not much better than the ordinary person on the street. The only group found to differ were philosophers, who were consistently more proficient than any of the other groups studied [65]. The problem caused by the enthymematic nature of the arguments was managed by applying the standard 'principle of charity' – that is, the hidden premises necessary to make the argument deductively valid were assumed.

The second problem, however, raises special theoretical difficulties when the subject-matter is moral reasoning, because there is no agreement on the appropriate formalisation of even first order deontic logic [66]. This lack of agreement is caused by the fact that a logic containing classic propositional logic, the ought operator Ox (read as 'it ought to be the case that x'), the possibility operator Cx (read as 'it can be the case that x') and the intuitively appealing axioms $Ox \Rightarrow Cx$ (ought implies can) and Oa and $Ob \Rightarrow O(a \text{ and } b)$ (if it ought to be the case that a and ought to be the case that b, then it ought to be the case that a and b (agglomeration)) must lead to the rejection of the existence of true moral dilemmas (that is, situations where an agent ought to do both a and b but can only do one of these) or to the rejection of one of the two axioms. This can be shown in the following way:

(I)   Oa .

(II)   Ob

(III)   Not C(a and b)

from I and II using agglomeration

(IV)   O(a and b)

from IV using ought implies can

(V)   C(a and b)

But now there is an obvious contradiction between III and V. We can therefore either reject the existence of true moral dilemmas as described in premise I–III or we can deny either the agglomeration rule or the ought implies can rule. Neither of these three approaches seems particularly attractive, although each has it advocates [see, for instance, the papers in 67, 68]. Another approach is to try to enrich the deontic logic by the introduction of quantificational, modal, and temporal resources. These attempts seem to lead to new paradoxes, and a full discussion would not be appropriate for the present purposes, since there are equally strong disagreements among proponents of the different 'enriched' deontic logics.

The implication of this discussion for the present study is that any attempt to assess the adequacy of the logical structure

of the ethical arguments presented by the respondents is problematic because there is genuine disagreement about the correct logical standard to use in such an assessment.

The perceptual construction of the moral problem

I have used the word 'attention', which I borrow from Simone
Weil, to express the idea of a just and loving gaze directed upon
an individual reality. I believe this to be the characteristic and
proper mark of the active moral agent. [2, p. 34]

The first step in the resolution of an ethical problem is that a
given situation is identified as a problem, and that the problem is further identified *as an ethical problem* (or at least as
containing ethically relevant features). Unless this task is
accomplished no ethical reasoning will ensue. If the problem
is identified as a problem, but not as an ethical problem, ethical considerations may still play some part, but they will be
seen as tangential to the real issue.

Moral philosophy has traditionally been relatively unin-
terested in the problem of moral sensitivity or moral perception, but literary writers have recognised it for a long time:

'I am far from attributing any part of Mr. Bingley's conduct to
design,' said Elizabeth; 'but without scheming to do wrong, or to
make others unhappy, there may be error, and there may be
misery. Thoughtlessness, want of attention to other people's feelings, and want of resolution, will do the business.' [69, p. 132]

Recently, a number of moral philosophers have become interested in the subject and have tried to redress this neglect. The
main points made in this new discussion are, first, that moral
perception is not a passive function but an active scanning of
the environment, and second, that one can be just as blame-
worthy for not seeing an ethical problem, as for not respond-
ing appropriately once one has seen it. To support the last
point, Lawrence Blum offers the following example:

John and Joan are sitting riding on a subway train. There are no
empty seats and some people are standing; yet the subway car is
not packed so tightly as to be uncomfortable for everyone. One of

the passengers standing is a woman in her thirties holding two relatively full shopping bags. John is not particularly paying attention
to the woman, but he is cognizant of her.

Joan by contrast, is distinctly aware that the woman is uncomfortable. ...

But the moral significance of the difference between John's and
Joan's perception of the situation lies not only in the relation
between that perception and the taking of beneficent action. It lies
in the fact of perception itself. ... That is to say, a morally significant aspect of the situation facing John fails to be salient for him,
and this is a defect in his character – perhaps not a very serious
moral defect, but a defect nevertheless. He misses something of the
moral reality confronting him. [70, pp. 702–4]

What is wrong here is not that John does not offer his seat to
the woman with the shopping bags, but that the thought never
enters his mind because of his deficient moral perception. Most
health care personnel have probably experienced similar situations, where they themselves have overlooked important ethical features, or where they have felt that colleagues have
acted in this way.

Some of the specific features of our ethical perception may
be innate. Hans Jonas has, for instance, argued that it is much
easier to perceive evil than to perceive good:

Because this is the way we are made: the perception of the *malum*
is infinitely easier to us than the perception of the *bonum*; it is more
direct, more compelling, less given to differences of opinion or
taste, and, most of all, obtruding itself without our looking for it.
An evil forces its perception on us by its mere presence, whereas
the beneficial can be present unobtrusively and remain unper-
ceived, unless we reflect on it (for which we must have special
cause). [71, p. 27]

But even if Jonas is right on a general level, it is probably the
case that much of our ethical perception requires training and
knowledge to function. This is pointed out by Iris Murdoch,
who notes that:

Of course virtue is good habit and dutiful action. But the background condition of such habit and such action, in human beings,

is a just mode of vision and a good quality of consciousness. It is a *task* to come to see the world as it is. [2, p. 91, emphasis in original]

A deep understanding of any field of human activity (painting, for instance) involves an increasing revelation of degrees of excellence and often a revelation of there being in fact little that is very good and nothing that is perfect. Increasing understanding of human conduct operates in a similar way. We come to perceive scales, distances, standards, and may incline to see as less than excellent what previously we were prepared to 'let by'. [2, p. 61]

In what follows I will mainly look at factors that influence ethical perception in a negative way. This emphasis is chosen because the analysis showed that it was very difficult to isolate positive factors influencing ethical perception, whereas negative factors were more easily identifiable. It may be that the positive factors are more person-specific.

Problems of ethical perception

The analysis of the interviews show that there are at least six different ways in which a specific situation can fail to be identified as an ethical problem.

1. It can be the case that the situation does not contain any features which make ethical reasoning relevant – that is, the situation is not an ethical problem. In this case the identification is correct, but, as I show below, such situations can be misidentified as ethical problems.

2. The observer can be insensitive to the ethically relevant features (the defect in moral perception described by Blum above).

3. The situation can contain ethically relevant features, but these are outweighed in saliency by other non-ethical features of the situation – that is, if there is an ethical problem, it is banal and it is therefore not identified as such. Or a problem is initially identified as some other kind of problem, and this identification pre-empts the identification as an ethical problem.

4. The situation can contain ethical features which will normally be taken to constitute an ethical problem, but because this problem has a firm solution in the mind of the person in the situation, no problem is identified.
5. Work pressure may block perception.
6. In some work settings it is seen as psychologically necessary not to see all problems.

All of these ways in which ethical perception might fail will be discussed in the following sections.

Framing effects in ethical perception

In the interviews it is possible to identify instances in which the respondents see ethical problems in situations where the most relevant understanding of the problem is as a technical problem. This is especially clear in the responses to case 1, which describes a double-blind placebo-controlled pharmaceutical trial, where the experimental drug has a clear and obvious side-effect: it causes a metallic taste in the mouth of a substantial proportion of those who take the drug.

The most obvious problem in this scenario is that the trial is seriously flawed methodologically. It is almost impossible to perform a double-blind trial if one of the arms of the trial has obvious side-effects that are identifiable by the patients (unless you can find a placebo with exactly the same side-effect). Nevertheless only six respondents identify this problem. Most of the other respondents either think that there are no problems because they will mention this side-effect in their consent form (not noticing that this will finally invalidate the study from a methodological point of view), or they think that there is an ethical problem about whether the side-effect should be mentioned or not.

This indicates that there must be a significant framing effect. In the context of the interview, the problem area is defined as ethics. When the respondents reach this case they have all been talking about ethics for more than half an hour, and they therefore try to identify ethical problems, even in situations where it requires quite some effort to overlook an extremely salient technical problem.

The existence of this framing effect has implications for ethical perception in daily health care work, since it is likely that the reverse effect also exists (that is, that ethical problems may be overlooked if the context defines the problem as technical).

If professional culture supports the initial presumption that a patient management problem is a technical problem, this framing of the problem may in itself make ethical factors more difficult to perceive.

One problem, one label

Ethical aspects of a situation may not be perceived as such because the situation has already acquired a label as some other kind of problem (e.g., technical, economic, administrative, legal). This mechanism is exemplified in the responses to case 9, about an elderly man operated on for cancer of the testis who has not been adequantely informed prior to discharge, and where the department has a huge backlog of discharge letters to general practitioners so that the GP will not be able to inform the man properly when he turns up. The respondents label this problem as a practical or administrative problem and the possible ethical components are not discussed.

Another example of the mechanism can be seen in case 6, describing an elderly man with cancer of the prostate and bronchitis, who is admitted to hospital with a severe attack of bronchitis, where it is discussed whether a no-resuscitation and no-respiratory-support order should be entered in his charts. Here the problem whether such an order is appropriate is seen as a purely technical problem to be decided by an assessment of the patient's medical state. Many respondents also identify an ethical problem in whether the man should be told about this decision. But this is seen as separate from the 'purely' technical decision.

External factors and ethical perception

External factors play a large role in modifying ethical perception. The main ones to influence ethical perception in a negative way are busyness and communication problems. Busyness influences ethical perception in several ways. It decreases the time spent with each individual patient, and thereby decreases the opportunity to perceive ethical problems. It tempts the professional to look for an easy fix (which will often be a solution taking only technical issues into account); and it makes it more difficult to communicate with the patient and other professionals.

The respondents also mention lack of communication and coordination as major obstacles to the identification of ethical problems. Several members of staff may hold individual bits of information, which, if put together, would reveal an ethical problem. But if the organisation is not designed to bring these people together, the difficulty will remain unnoticed. General practitioners have a special difficulty in this regard, because they often become aware of problems which occurred during a patient's hospitalisation and which are still unresolved. In these cases they have to consider whether it is 'worth their while' to make the hospital department aware of the problem, or whether they should try to solve it themselves.

Internal factors and ethical perception

Internal factors may also play a role in ethical perception. A person's self-interest may in some cases block the perception of an ethical problem, but it may also in some cases make ethical problems more easily perceivable. This is illustrated by responses to case 3, in which a pharmaceutical company wants to make yet another comparison between two NSAIDs (ibuprofen, naproxen, aspirin, etc.). It is explicitly stated in the case description that this trial has very little scientific value, and that it is mainly done in order to get a new, but not more effective, drug on the market. Most respondents claim that there are no ethical problems in this case, because they would just reject an offer from the pharmaceutical company to participate. This rejection is, however, often qualified in the case of junior doctors, who state that their position would depend on whether a consultant at their department was interested in the study. One interpretation of this finding is that the ethical perception and decision in this case partly depend on how much the professional personally stands to gain or lose.

Routinisation of ethical perception

All the physicians and nurses interviewed worked in clinical departments or in general practice, and had daily contact with patients. It is therefore reasonable to assume that they had to experience ethical problems now and again. Studies of the frequency of ethical problems indicate that they occur in relation to about 20 per cent of all in-patients in a department of internal medicine, and in at least 5 per cent of all patient encounters in a casualty department [72, 73]. These figures were arrived at by letting physicians themselves identify the ethical problems, and the numbers must therefore be seen as minimum estimates. This means that even if a health care professional sees only fifty different patients each week, there is a fairly good chance that he or she will encounter an ethically problematic situation every week.[1]

It could therefore be expected that all the people interviewed would have been able to give a relevant answer to the first question in the interview: 'Tell me about the last ethical problem you experienced in your work?' This was not, however, the case. Most of the respondents could point to a specific situation, but a few were unable to do so. How can this finding be explained?

An explanation can perhaps be found if we look at one of the examples of this phenomenon:[2]

I: *I would like to start with you trying to tell me about the latest ethical problem you think you have met in your clinical work.*

R: *That is difficult because you don't go around collecting ethical problems. And in the final analysis you solve problems, so it is really somewhat difficult. So I have tried, after we have talked together, to think some things through, but it is a strangely backwards way of doing it in the final analysis and – yes, I don't really know what I found out last time I thought about it; well, one thing you always can discuss is, to what degree you should tell patients all about their illness. On that issue there are some guidelines from the Board of Health and other official bodies. In practice it can be somewhat dif-*

ficult to administer these things, and you can also sometimes wish to speculate, how appropriate it is – Now, I am mainly concerned with cardiac patients, where it is maybe not as dramatic. But the patients I meet now and again, who have a malignant disease, there the situation is somewhat different, and there, in some places, if we take especially malignant diseases, they always tell them what they are suffering from. That can sometimes lead to problems for those who receive it, they are left in a vacuum, and in previous times where you had a firm idea that if you behave in the right way, there was continued life on the other side, like in Bach's cantata and Brorson's psalms. Now the situation is not so, for most people – and because of that it can be very difficult for those people to get on after that – and therefore you can wonder, whether it is really appropriate to say it. And we in the department tend to have the view that if the patients ask about it and seem generally interested in having an answer, then they get an answer, but otherwise we don't necessarily tell it. There can be special circumstances, if, for instance, there are family matters that are necessary to settle, that can lead to a change in attitude, but those are some of the things one can discuss.

[...]

I: *Do you feel that you meet any other kind of problems, which you would call ethical problems?*

R: *Well, in the final analysis it is somewhat of a rationalisation. Sometimes you meet the problem, which again is not always a problem, but it is a question of how you manage the case, and we have in our department met the attitude that problems should really be solved and thought through in advance, and it should not be something, you leave to the single individual to find out. There can be a problem, that is to continue treatment of very ill patients, and in the department we have the point of view that we take the matter to a conference. And that is also due to the Hilden case, where a single man was left with the responsibility. So we take it to a conference and discuss whether it is a situation where you should say, that in case of cardiac arrest no resuscitation should be attempted, and if complications arise how actively should one treat, so there are some guidelines – so again, in so far as we have a procedure in that area, it represents a problem to that degree, because, other things being equal, if there are diverging opinions, then we say that the patients should have the truth.*

[...]

I: *Do you think that you meet any more general ethical problems –*

that is, problems which are not directly concerned with the treatment of the individual patient?

R: *Well, this is again difficult to answer – I don't dare really to answer, because you decide on a concrete case and you find a solution. If you don't have a solution – well, then you don't speculate much more about it.*

I: *So for you it is – now you are saying that if you have a solution, you don't speculate about it – so is an ethical problem a problem, where it is difficult to find a solution?*

R: *Well, in so far as you yourself say that it is a problem, then it is something which has not found its solution in the last instance in some way – but issues can still arise which you then have to consider specifically.*

[...]

I: *Do you think that you see most of the questions you ought to see?*

R: *In so far as I don't think that there are any major ethical problems floating around, I don't think that the problems are so big.* (DSM)

What characterises this long quote is, first, that although ethical problems are mentioned, they are not personalised. Neither the physician answering, nor any identifiable patient occurs in the descriptions of the problems. The problems are presented as abstract and theoretical, where the type of problem (e.g., truth-telling) is seen as important, but without any contextual features. The respondent does not really answer the question 'try to tell me about the latest ethical problem you think you have met in your clinical work'; he answers a question more like 'what kind of ethical problems have you heard or thought about recently?'.

The second characteristic is that legal considerations and pronouncements of the Board of Health are seen as main causes of the problems. That is, the first ethical problem described is not what patients should be told from an ethical point of view, but how guidelines from the Board of Health can be implemented without too much trouble.

The key to understanding the failure to recount real personal ethical problems is probably to be found in the two sentences '*If you don't have a solution – well, then you don't speculate much more about it.*' and '*Well, in so far as you your-self say, that it is a problem, then it is something which has not found its solution in the last instance in some way.*' Taken at face value, these two statements would imply that 'permanent' ethical problems do not occur. The first statement implies that problems which do not have a solution are pushed to the back of the mind, and the second that situations that do have a solution are not problems. A problem can therefore only exist as a problem for a limited period of time – either it is solved and disappears, or it is not solved within a reasonable time-span and is then discounted. The solution to a solved problem may of course enter the store of stock solutions to various types of ethical problems, but when the same type of problem is encountered again, it will be as a type of problem, and not as an individual problem. The explanation for the lack of identi-fication of any personally experienced ethical problem in this case therefore seems to involve two distinct components: first, a routinisation of ethics, where recurring ethical problems are seen as already solved and therefore not as problems, and second, a discounting of unsolvable problems.

The second component is clearly problematic, since it is presumably the difficult problems that require the most thought and the most diligent attention. It is, however, an atti-tude toward ethical problems which is also mentioned by sev-eral other respondents.

Whether the first of these components constitutes a defi-ciency in ethical perception mainly depends on how complex ethical problems really are. If it is the case that they can be easily typecast, and that solutions are transferable within each type (e.g., within the type 'truth-telling'), there is no problem. If, however, the features of each individual case play a major role in ethical decisions, there is a problem. In that case it is not sufficient just to refer the case to a given type, and use the solution for that type. The type-solution may give a first approximation to the individual solution, but ethical reasoning must be applied to see whether it is really the solution that fits the individual case. There is little doubt that many (most?) ethical problems are of the second kind described, where indi-

vidual features matter, and a routinisation of ethical perception is therefore unfortunate, because it hides ethically relevant factors from view. A routinisation of ethical perception
will, almost inevitably, lead to a routinisation of ethical decision-making. This is a problem if the rules of thumb that are
developed are not sufficiently sensitive to contextual features.

That routinisation of ethical perception and decision-
making is a common phenomenon receives some support from
Davis's study of ethical dilemmas in nursing, which shows that
younger nurses perceived that they had more ethical dilemmas
in their daily work than did older nurses. This finding could
either be explained by routinisation, by ethical burn-out (see
next section), or by a simple cohort effect [74].

Interpersonal variation in ethical perception

A semi-quantitative analysis of the responses given to the thirteen case-studies presented in the interview substantiates that
there are large differences in perceptions of ethical problems.
Some respondents saw one or more ethical problems in all thirteen cases and some only in seven or eight of them. There are
also great differences in perceptions when different cases are
compared. All respondents identified ethical problems in case
5 (colleague has made error and harmed patient) and case 7
(elderly patient with congestive heart failure and pneumonia,
family states that 'they wish that no theraputic measures
should be taken if an exacerbation occurs'), but less than a
third found any ethical problem in case 3 (trial where a pharmaceutical company wants to make yet another comparison
between two NSAIDs) and only about half found ethical problems in case 11 (operation of HIV-positive patient).

Because of the non-representative sample the figures should
not be given too much weight except as broad indications of
tendencies. The finding of great individual differences in the
ethical perceptions of health care professionals is consistent
with findings from a number of other studies.

Hébert et al. found large differences in the number of ethical
issues medical students could identify in clinical vignettes
describing ethical problems [75]. Their expert panel identified

between 7 and 9 ethical issues in each vignette, and their student respondents (only) managed to identify an average of 2.72 per vignette, within a range of 0–7 issues. The authors mention that they found a normal distribution both for the whole sample and for each separate class of students investigated. Keller found, as mentioned above, that out of 6 dilemma situations a sample of nurses only identified an average of 2.7 as dilemmas, within a range of 0–6 [32]. Stevens and McCormick studied participants in a multi-disciplinary, postgraduate ethics course [76]. They found that the students' ability to identify ethical issues in a given case increased from an average of 2.4 issues before case discussions to 3.6 after the discussions.

The existence of general differences of ethical perception – described as a threshold phenomenon is well known by the respondents who experience the differences in their daily contact with colleagues. Some people have lower thresholds for calling something an ethical problem:

> *There are some who are very ethically oriented and who see problems or evaluations and factors in everything, and then there are others who appear as if they are walking around with blinkers. And in this department we have some who are walking around with blinkers in a class of their own.* (DIM)

> *I only see those where I myself am in doubt. Then there are others who can have their doubts, where I think I have a firm opinion about the matter. So, there are undoubtedly others who can disagree with me in some of my actions, who will see it as ethical problems, where I think – well, where I think that is the way it should be done, we usually do it this way, so let's do it this way.* (DIM)

It is difficult to see any way to specify the optimal threshold in practical terms, and therefore hard to distinguish between those who are optimally aware of ethical problems, those who perceive too few, and those who perceive too many. The analysis in the present and the preceding sections does, however, indicate that all three kinds of person can be found in the health care system.

It is perhaps paradoxical to state that too many ethical problems can be perceived. Is it not a good thing to perceive all the ethical problems one encounters? An answer to this question must have two sides. Yes, it is good not to overlook any ethical problems. No, it is bad to take all ethical problems very seriously. In the health care setting there are so many ethical problems that some must be solved by applying simple rules of thumb. It is both psychologically and practically impossible to deal with all problems through formal deliberation. The task of the health care professional is therefore to navigate between the Scylla of neglecting all problems, and the Charybdis of taking all problems very seriously. There is probably no precise rule which can describe exactly where the right balancing point is, but given that we have some ideas about the seriousness of various ethical problems, we can, at least, see when too many serious problems are being neglected.

The reasons for the identified differences in ethical perception are manifold (including the routinisation described above), but one of the more worrying processes which the respondents describe is what could be called ethical burn-out. This is the situation where health care professionals simply stop identifying ethical problems, because there are too many to cope with:

> Yes, I think, I think that you can have periods where you, like, choose to say, well, I can't handle the ethical, now I just have to do it like it is. (DSF)

> Well, when you work, well, you have to, a psychiatric admissions ward in a socially deprived area like this, you have a long list of routines, and if you saw all ethical problems, you would probably have consciously to overlook many. (DSM)

The risk of ethical burn-out is clearly connected to the level of pressure and the amount of work, and to the organisational issues discussed in Chapter 5.

The construction of ethical problems

In the previous sections I have talked about ethical perception in a way that is similar to how I could have talked about the perception of physical objects in the world. This way of talking is useful, but it is not the whole story about ethical perception. Ethical problems are not only perceived, they are also to a significant degree constructed.

When I see an ethical problem, I always see a specific ethical problem. The statement 'I can see that I have an ethical problem, but I wonder what it is' sounds strange. Ethical problems are specified from the first moment. This specification may be wrong, and I may later change my opinion about what kind of ethical problem I have, but this does not change the fact that the problem was specified in some way from the beginning.

The initial specification is not something that is immediately perceivable. Ethical problems do not present themselves to the senses like the colour or shape of an object, they are constructed by inference from a range of features in the situation. This construction is influenced by the contextual features in the situation, and also by the personal characteristics of health care professionals, and by the organisation of health care.

This is clearly illustrated in the responses to the cases used in the interview, where many of the respondents felt that they had to complete the context in various ways, before they could reach a decision. The mechanism is illustrated by the following short initial response to case 6, a case describing an elderly man with cancer of the prostate and bronchitis, who is admitted to hospital with a severe attack of bronchitis, and where a decision is being contemplated about whether or not to offer respiratory support or resuscitation:

> *You can live several years with a cancer of the prostate, even if you have single metastases to the spinal column. Here I would probably say that if his level of function is at about grade 1, then he should be put in a respirator, and maybe also if he is in grade 2. But if he is grade 3 and has a malignant disease, he should not if he was in functional group 3, even if he did not have a malignant disease. So this question must be graded. His malignant disease should not decide whether he is put in a respirator. That should be decided by his functional level when he is well — that is, without pulmonary disease, except the chronic.* (DSM)

The context that is filled in here is the technical context (that is, the exact severity of the patient's disease), but in other examples it is the social context (e.g., relationship to family, etc.) or the personal context (e.g., what does the patient really want):

> *There is a range of problems that can be uncovered by getting more information. So again, you should not react in a very rigid way, but you have to get some information, you have to have knowledge about the patient, about the relatives, about your staffing level etc., etc., so there are many ethical problems in this as well.* (DSM)

These contextual features not only change the solution of the problem, they also change the way the problem is perceived. The importance given to the unique contextual features in every situation can be so great that it leads to the conclusion that moral knowledge is not transferable between situations (that is, an extreme ethical particularism), or to the more moderate conclusion reached by most respondents that although ethical rules can act as rules of thumb, every situation has to be evaluated in its particularity:

> *I firmly believe that it has, yes, I believe that it is supporting if you have been in a situation before which reminds you of this one, or whether you are totally new to it. Because you always reflect on these decisions afterwards, a kind of post-reflection. You can learn from them, but there is, I think, nevertheless, something special about every situation you can put on top of it. It is like two layers.* (NIF)

Surprising constructions of case-studies

That ethical problems are constructed and are not immediately perceivable is perhaps most clearly demonstrated in those cases, where the respondents present a truly aberrant and surprising construction of the problem. By surprising I mean a construction that seems to take no account of the ethical problem which most people would see as salient in a given case. Surprising constructions can therefore only be easily identified in response to case-studies describing some fairly clear ethical problem.

In this study I have found some examples of surprising constructions, and closer analysis reveals some interesting features about the influence of context and ethical theory on ethical perception. I will analyse three such examples, showing how ethical perception is shaped by personal experience, a specific role in the organisation, and the ethical theory of the person.

In response to case 8 which describes a situation in which two people with cardiac arrest arrive almost simultaneously at the casualty ward where the respondent is the only qualified professional, and where the superior has gone home to sleep, the following conclusion was presented by a junior physician:

> *But it is like, I can imagine that what this is about is that whether or not you should call the superior in could be something ethical, and at the same time two patients are coming in, and I think that there is no discussion about it – if there are no others than him, he should be called in* (DIF)

And a consultant psychiatrist offered the following observation, as the first statement in a longer argument:

> *There are no ethical problems in the fact that the superior is on his way home. The superior should of course be contacted and come in as quickly as possible.* (DSM)

The normal construction of this problem is that the ethical problem consists in the fact that it is very difficult to treat the two patients at the same time, and that a choice may have to be made to try to resuscitate only one of them (this was also the end result of the argument by the psychiatrist quoted here). The 'normal' problem is, should I choose to treat only one, and if so which one? (In fact, many of the respondents spent quite a long time explaining why the situation would not happen in real life, so that they would not have to make this choice.)

The difficulty that is pushed to the foreground by the junior doctor in this case is obviously a problem, and this is underscored by the presence of the consideration in the argument of the consultant psychiatrist. Bluntly stated, the problem is as follows: should I annoy my superior by calling him back to work or should I just try to handle things on my own and be a good and efficient subordinate? One may question whether this is really an ethical problem, or 'only' a prudential problem, but it is perhaps more illuminating to ask why it becomes so salient that the more 'normal' construction of the problem is blocked out.

If the whole interview is taken into account it is evident that the junior doctor in question is very much aware of ethical problems in her daily work, and that she is able to reason well about them. There is no evidence of a 'general' defect of ethical perception or reasoning. Thus there is a temptation just to dismiss her response to this case as idiosyncratic and unexplainable, but that way out is too easy. In the interview there are two other sections which may help in finding an explanation for the surprising construction:

> But you are brought up with the idea, that the decisions made by a senior registrar and a consultant are the valid ones. And it is no use, when you are in a locum lasting 1, 2, or 3 months, it is no use shouting too loudly, because then your job isn't extended; and I think that many keep a very low profile, and I have done that as well in some places, because you have to do it, you don't want to be awkward. (DIF)

> Part of the problem is also, I think, that some places are very busy, there you have to, you do not have the time to mess around with something, you have to make a decision and get on with it, because there are four more lying and waiting, so it has to be this way. (DIF)

These sections indicate that this particular junior doctor has had some negative experiences with the pressure to conform in a hierarchical structure and with the demands for instant decision-making. These prior experiences make her construction of the case understandable, although they do not give us a watertight causal explanation. In this context it is also interesting that she refers to the senior registrar as 'him' since no gendered terms were used in the case.

The second set of surprising constructions occurred in response to a case about a patient who has been seeing the health care professional over a long period of time. He presents himself with visual problems and asks for the name of a good ophthalmologist. The initial investigation shows that his visual acuity is far below the legal limit for driving a motor vehicle:

Yes, in this system we are in principle not allowed to recommend doctors or recommend further measures from the social system, where money is involved. In some cases you are, luckily, so ignorant that, as a matter of fact, you don't know the practising ophthalmologists, in this case it is an ophthalmologist, then the problem is solved, because you cannot. But the problem is, if you actually have the knowledge, then it can be very difficult to say that 'I am not allowed to tell you'. Most probably find a way to tell it anyway in the specific case, since it is not all patients who come asking for an ophthalmologist. Just because one patient comes asking about this specific problem will not lead to the ophthalmologist suddenly having many more clients or patients. So I am certain that I would manage to tell the patient who I think they ought to contact, but I am not allowed to do it.(NSM)

If the patient's vision is very poor he could get in trouble by driving a car. What you can explain to him is that it seems like he has trouble orientating himself, so the most sensible thing to do would be to take a new consultative driving test to see whether he is at all capable of driving a car. Because it would be a pity for him, if he were to drive the car and get into trouble, and happen to kill somebody or hurt himself or somebody else, and he would then probably be sorry. Therefore it is most sensible to have a test to see whether or not he can drive his car. (DGF)

The 'normal' construction of this case is that the problem consists in the conflict between a legal and moral obligation to prevent the patient from driving a motor vehicle, and the considerations of his well-being and the importance of maintaining a positive relationship with him.

The first of these constructions was presented by a chief nurse, who throughout the interview displayed a keen sense of the problems nurses have by being 'wedged' between doctors and patients. For him, the problem becomes whether his moral responsibility to help the patient can be discharged within the institutional constraints imposed on employees in the public health care system.

The second aberrant construction was presented by a general practitioner. What is surprising here is not the result, or the form of the argument, but the main ethical premise leading to the result:

Because it would be a pity for him if he were to drive the car and get into trouble, and happen to kill somebody or hurt himself or somebody else, and he would then probably be sorry. (DGF)

The most likely explanation of what is, happening here is that the respondent holds an ethical theory stating that in ethical problems concerning the patients the paramount consideration is the best interest or well-being of the patient, and any decision has to be explained in terms of this consideration.

The problem is therefore framed exclusively in terms of how the different outcomes might affect the patient. The respondent probably 'knows' that the right decision is to make sure that the patient does not drive, but, given the constraints the theory sets for acceptable premises, she is forced to posit serious psychological damage to the patient if he kills or harms somebody else, to make the conclusion 'right'. For most people the wrongness in killing would be localised in what happens to the person being killed, and not in what effect the killing has on the killer, This construction exemplifies how the perception of an ethical problem is influenced/determined by the ethical theory of the perceiver.

The importance of context in the perception of ethical problems and the presence of truly surprising constructions also presents a methodological problem for empirical research using questionnaires based on such case-studies. We like to believe that the respondents' answers are based on a straightforward interpretation of the case presented in the questionnaire, but this may not always be so. Respondents may construct their own different accounts of the problem by adding whatever context they feel is appropriate to reach a solution, and since their answers will always be based on their own account, and not on the account of the researcher, the exact interpretation of the answers may be difficult.

Individual components of the professional ethical framework

The initial analysis and open coding of the interviews gave rise to the following categories of statements occurring in ethical arguments:

1. Statements referring to consequences:
   what is best for the patient a) in a technical sense, b) in an ethical sense, c) in a social sense;
   what is best for the patient's family;
   what is best for society;
   what is best for the department or individual colleagues.
2. Statements referring to rights/duties/obligations of the patient or the health care professional:
   ethical;
   legal.
3. Statements referring to respect for the patient.
4. Statements referring to relationships with the patient.

The two first categories of statement (with subcategories) match the traditional divide in moral philosophy between consequentialist and deontological theories, whereas the last two categories are not easy to fit into the traditional scheme.

Respect for the patient is seen as something the patient is owed in virtue of being a human being. Carers have an obligation to respect the patient which does not depend on the characteristics of the patient, or the relationship between patient and carer. This respect is mainly seen as an attitude or disposition that the carer ought to have, and which only secondarily gives rise to any actions. That is, both *having respect* and *showing respect* are seen as important. The attitude of respect or the disposition to respect will of course have some implications for action. It will block depersonalisation of the patient and disrespectful treatment, and it will create courtesy and understanding. These actions are valuable, but it is not only the actions that make having respect important. It is therefore reasonable to subdivide respect into two subcategories: respect(act) and respect(virtue). Here, respect(virtue) describes that part of the respect concept that is involved when it is assessed whether individual actions display proper respect, whereas respect(act) describes the part of respect that is concerned with directly respectful actions. This idea about the importance of respect for the patient could, with some difficulty, be subsumed under the categories of traditional moral philosophy, if it was not seen as a theory-given aim (that is, seen not to belong to the part of the theory producing moral evaluation of actions), but as part of (one of) the best set(s) of desires or attitudes or dispositions prescribed by the theory (that is, seen to belong to the part of the theory evaluating agents) [77]. For analytic purposes it is, however, better to keep respect as two separate categories, one concerned with the disposition and one concerned with directly respectful acts.

The statements referring to relationships with the patient talk about the importance of creating and maintaining a relationship in three different ways: as a means to obtain good ends, as directly producing good in people's lives, and as an end in itself. The first of these views is clearly exemplified when psychiatrists talk about the 'therapeutic alliance' as a necessary precondition for successful treatment, and in situations where professionals evaluate 'strange requests' from patients (e.g., from Jehova's Witnesses not to have blood transfusions). In the latter type of case it is seen as essential to create a relationship with the patient which makes it possible to assess the rationale behind the request and the 'depth of conviction'. The second view is also quite easy to understand. It seems incontrovertible that having relationships with other people is one of the things that creates good in people's lives. These two views on the importance of relationships can easily be subsumed in a consequentialist framework.

The third view claims that relationships are important neither as a means to something else, nor because they produce good in the life of people, but simply because creating or maintaining a relationship is a good thing in itself. In the data it is not possible to distinguish whether what is good is the creation or maintenance of relationships (the activity/process), or the mere fact that relationships are created and maintained (the result). This point of view is very difficult to fit into a deontological or consequentialist model, but it does have connections to an ethic of care, where the caring relationship is seen as valuable in itself, and it could also be conceptualised as a virtue. The relationship category was therefore subdivided into two subcategories: relationship(act) falling under the general category of consequences for the patient and including statements referring to relationships as a means to good ends or as a producer of good, and relationship(virtue) including statements about relationships as an end in themselves. In what follows, when I refer to relationships and respect it is in the sense of relationship(virtue) and respect(virtue).

The only category of statements in which there is any appreciable difference between nurses and doctors is that which refers to the importance of creating and maintaining relationships with patients. Nurses speak more eloquently about this subject than doctors, not only when they recount their own ethical problems, but also when they respond to the cases that were presented during the interview. The simplest explanation for this difference is that it is a function of their working conditions, as it is both easier and more necessary for nurses to establish relationships with patients. This explanation is somewhat supported by the finding that within the group of doctors interviewed general practitioners and psychiatrists also speak more about the importance of relationships with patients.

Within the group of statements referring to rights, duties, and obligations, many individual rights are mentioned: the patient has a right to life, to decide about his or her own treatment, to have an advance directive respected, to be told the truth, not to be told more than he or she wants to be told, and to compensation for iatrogenic injury. The professional has a duty to maintain confidentiality, to be honest, to tell the truth, to obey the law, to inform other professionals, to help people in need (including an assumption of a certain level of personal risk), and to uphold justice with regard to age, social status, etc. Although the content of each individual duty is important in its own right, it is more important for the understanding of ethical reasoning to look at the scope and justification of the duties.

The duties and rights identified here are not seen as

absolute; all of them (with the possible exception of the right to be told the truth) can be superseded by other considerations. This is illustrated by the responses to case 10 about an elderly man admitted with pneumonia, who is confused at night, disturbs the other patients, and refuses to take a sleeping pill. In the analysis of this situation most respondents weigh the man's legal and moral right to refuse treatment against the harm he is causing other patients and the resources he drains from the department. A few then decide to try to give him something against his will (in principle illegal), whereas most decide to respect his wishes. But the mere fact that the decision is analysed in this way shows that the patient's right to decide about his own treatment is not seen as absolute. When I use words such as 'weigh' or 'balance' it does not imply that the respondents necessarily use some common underlying metric. A more correct description would probably be that they look at two possible outcomes and choose one of them, claiming that it is the better, but without claiming that choosing this action is at the same time the right thing to do. A similar balancing is prominent in the responses to case 12, where a legal duty to report a patient as dangerous in traffic is weighed against the best interests of the patient.

With regard to justification there is a distinction between legal and ethical justifications, and for almost all of the rights and duties mentioned here both types are mentioned. As the responses to case 10 show neither a legal nor an ethical justification for a right to make decisions about one's own treatment makes it an absolute right.

The technical and the ethical

A prominent feature in the ethical reasoning of health care professionals is the frequent reference to technical/medical knowledge. This is not surprising, since this knowledge is necessary in many situations in order to reach the appropriate ethical solution. Unfortunately, it is not always the case that the best technical solution (what is best for the patient in a technical sense) and the best ethical solution (what is best for the patient in an ethical sense) coincide. It is therefore necessary to distinguish between the ethically best, and the technically best, but this distinction is not always realised by health care professionals. Some conflate the two:

> *So it is, how shall I put it, a medical technical question about, what you can do in a specific situation which sets the limits.* (DSM)
>
> *If you can keep the standard high and say, I try to give my patients the best possible treatments, you have good ethics.* (DIM)

This conflation is often innocuous in its actual effects on the treatment of the patient, but it is insidious with regard to ethical reasoning because it distorts the reasoning process, and leaves the health care professional with a misleading picture of the extent to which technical expertise can be equated with ethical expertise. The emphasis on technical considerations also entails that even though a problem has been correctly labelled as an ethical problem, it may still be considered in a purely technical way.

Professional ethical reasoning

To get a full understanding of the structure of the ethical reasoning of health care professionals it is necessary to fit the individual components into a larger framework.

Ross and prima facie duties

A simple way to supply this framework would be to adopt the ideas of the British philosopher W. D. Ross who in the 1930s, developed a theory of ethics built on an intuitionist metaethics. His normative ethics developed the claim that we have an irreducible number of different ethical duties, all of which are of a prima facie nature [41, 78], or in his own words:

> Any possible act has many sides to it which are relevant to its rightness or wrongness; it will bring pleasure to some people, pain to others; it will be keeping of a promise to one person, at the cost of being a breach of confidence to another, and so on. We are quite incapable of pronouncing straight off on its rightness or wrongness in the totality of these aspects; it is only by recognizing these different features one by one that we can approach the forming of a

judgement on the totality of its nature; our first look reveals these features in isolation, one by one; they are what appears *prima facie*. And secondly, they are *prima facie, obligations*. It is easy to be so impressed by the rightness of an act in one respect that we suppose it to be therefore necessarily the act we are bound to do. But an act may be right in one respect and wrong in more important respects, and therefore not, in the totality of its aspects, the most right of the acts open to us, and then we are not obliged to do it; and another act may be wrong in some respect and yet in its totality the most right of all the acts open to us, and then we *are* bound to do it. *Prima facie* obligation depends on some one aspect of the act; obligation or disobligation attaches to it in virtue of the totality of its aspects. [78, p. 84, emphasis in original]

For while an act may well be *prima facie* obligatory in respect of one character and *prima facie* forbidden in virtue of another, it becomes obligatory or forbidden only in virtue of the totality of its ethically relevant characteristics. [78, p. 86, emphasis in original]

What we have, according to Ross, are a number of prima facie duties, which are balanced against each other when we consider an ethical problem. There are no absolute duties, and there is no higher level of morality than prima facie duties (that is, when we have two conflicting prima facie duties, we cannot refer back to some more basic ethical principles to solve the conflict). When we solve an ethical problem, we decide that one of the prima facie duties is overriding in this situation, and that the conflicting prima facie duties are thereby seen not to be real duties in this situation.

If Ross's normative theory had been able to provide an adequate description of how the individual components of the ethical framework of health care professionals fit together, the analysis of the interviews could have ended here with a simple labelling of each identified component of the framework as a prima facie duty. There are, however, two features of the ethical reasoning of health care professionals that do not fit Ross's theory. The respondents see their reasoning as much more integrated than Ross describes it, and they do not believe that duties are automatically dissolved without remainder when they are overridden.

Grounded theory and the paradigm model

Because the Ross theory does not fit the data it is necessary to investigate whether a better account emerges from a further analysis of the data. It is in this stage of the process that grounded theory methodology becomes particularly useful. Through axial and selective coding, and use of the paradigm model described by Strauss and Corbin, it is possible to elucidate the connection between the categories one has generated during the phase of open coding [26]. The paradigm model is a tool for linking subcategories to categories through a set of relationships. Strauss's and Corbin's simplification of the model looks as follows [modified from 26, p. 99]:

causal conditions → phenomenon → context
→ intervening conditions → action/interaction strategies
→ consequences

What I tried in the initial axial coding of the ethical reasoning sections of the data was to 'fit a model', in which the causal conditions were subdivided into two parts; 'deep ethical framework' and 'ethical principles'; ethical reasoning and decision-making was the phenomenon; the features of the specific decision-making situation constituted the context; the organisational context created the intervening conditions; the choice of action was the strategy; and actual action was the consequence. It quickly became evident that this model was too simple. It left a lot of material unaccounted for, and other material could only be brought in with great difficulty. The attempt to fit this simple model did, however, make two things clear; first, that the notion of responsibility plays a significant role in the ethical framework of the health care professionals, and second, that a model really able to make sense of the data (provide the best explanation) cannot be linear, but will have to include feedback loops. At the end of this chapter I will return to a more realistic total model, but here I want to move on to the role played by the notion of responsibility.

The 'discovery' of 'protective responsibility'

One of the questions that had entered my interview guide during its development was 'Do health care professionals have a special ethical responsibility?'. Neither I, nor the people with whom I discussed the various versions of the guide, had seen this question as especially important. It was mainly included to act as a kind of introduction to the next question, which was 'Do you feel that your personal ethical thinking is typical within your professional group?'.

During the initial attempts at axial coding of the data on ethical reasoning, it did, nevertheless, become evident that the answers generated by this question about responsibility, and the other remarks about responsibility scattered throughout the interviews, were crucial for an understanding of how the individual ethical considerations mentioned by the respondents could be brought together in a larger coherent framework.

I started to work with responsibility as a presumptive core category, and to try to see whether this could explain the individual ethical considerations put forward, as well as the deviations from traditional moral philosophy, and the simultaneous use of consequentialist and deontological modes of reasoning.

By re-analysis of the category of 'responsibility', which had been identified during open coding, it became clear that it could be divided in two new categories. One of these was named 'professional responsibility' and is concerned with responsibilities which the profession as such has been given either through legislation, through a specific organisational role, or through formal internal ethical rules. The other new category was initially named 'personal responsibility' and later renamed 'protective responsibility'. This category contains material concerned with the responsibilities which the individual person acquires as a result of working in a health care setting.

Further analysis showed that a model with 'protective responsibility' as the core category is able to provide an adequate explanation of the ethical reasoning of the health care professionals studied here. It is interesting to note the connection between protective responsibility and the concept of medical responsibility identified in *Boys in White*, Becker's *et al.*'s seminal study of medical students. They describe medical responsibility in the following way:

> First, we must see that basically the term refers to the archetypal feature of medical practice: the physician who holds his patient's fate in his hands and on whom the patient's life or death may depend. Medical responsibility is responsibility for the patient's well-being, and the exercise of medical responsibility is seen as the basic and key action of the practising physician. The physician is most a physician when he exercises this responsibility. [79, p. 224]

Protective responsibility

As the name of the concept implies, 'protective responsibility' is a specific kind of responsibility, a responsibility to protect. This name was chosen because the data showed that the health care professionals linked their personal responsibility to the vulnerable state of the patients:

> *We get very close to the integrity-limit of individual people, people come in who are vulnerable, who are ill, who depend upon the fact that there is someone who can and will help them. That is why we have a special responsibility to do it in a decent and proper way, and to observe the ordinary rules for how we are together as people, and the ethical rules, the technical must be taken care of. We don't have, well it is people who come to us, and they have a problem which they really believe we want to help them with in some way.* (DIM)

Also mentioned as important are the often profound and irreversible effects of medical treatment:

> *The decisions of physicians are often, can be very decisive/important for other people – that is, for the further life of their patients. Because of this they have an obligation to be conscientious, and not just to try to secure the best possible opportunities and conditions for the patient, but also to try to protect the patient against the worst possible outcomes. That means that all professionals, yes, even a hairdresser, have similar problems, but at least for the hairdresser the consequences will never be as great, you can always let the hair grow out again.* (DIM)

When you meet the patient, you meet another human being who is vulnerable, who often trusts you, and whose life you can influence in a significant way. This creates a specific responsibility toward this other human being, which can be difficult to understand for outsiders, but which nevertheless plays a significant role in the deliberation of health care professionals. In their minds it is both related to the power they have, and to the respect they have to show:

> *You have an incredible power which you can misuse, and which can be misunderstood. So I definitely think that there is a — You can be in a special situation when you discuss with other people who are not doctors, who often have difficulty in understanding this way of thinking, or the problem you present.* (DIM)

> *You are working with a vulnerable group, a group which is in danger, which does not possess the same resources, and then you have to — It is people you are working with. There are considerations you have to take into account, you cannot view them as things, and there are other considerations than the purely economical. That is the reason why maybe all health care personnel ought to have some, ought to show that you have great ethical responsibility, because they are working with persons who are in crisis.* (NIF)

That the concept is called protective responsibility is furthermore intended to signify that it is primarily seen as a responsibility to protect from evil, and not, for instance, as a responsibility for the total well-being of the patient. The centrality of harm is exemplified in the following quote from a longer argument about the problem caused by a psychiatric patient who does not want to wash himself:

> *Because it must be the choice of the individual patient, 'I don't want to be washed now', that is the choice of the patient, but I can see that it is going to be dangerous for his health if I do not intervene now. And that is where I, as a professional, have to act. I can look so much ahead that I can see that it can become dangerous for the patient, either that the illness will not be healed, or in the case of a very ill patient, that you could be threatened.* (NIF)

The primary evil in the health care context is illness and disease, but protective responsibility also entails duties to protect

the patient against her or himself, against the family, against
the professionals, and against society.

The best way to display these features is by looking at one
specific ethical problem discussed by all respondents – that is,
'How much say should patients have in discussions about their
own treatment?' – because this problem brings into play many
of the individual ethical considerations identified above, as
well as many of the prominent players.

Protective responsibility and treatment decisions

The initial response to the question 'How much say should
patients have in discussions about their own treatment?', is,
without exception 'patients should always decide for themselves', but almost all respondents go on to qualify this, either
directly, or through their responses to the cases presented. The
right to decide is always understood as a negative right. The
patient has a right to refuse any treatment, but does not have
a right to demand a specific treatment. In some cases patients
will be given the treatment they demand, but only if the treatment is seen as acceptable by the professional. Some of the
older respondents also mention that this emphasis on respect
for autonomy represents a relatively recent shift in the ethics
of health care.

The main qualification of patients' unlimited autonomy is
where their best interests as seen by the professional, are seriously harmed by the choices they make. In these cases a
patient's rights and the consequences point to opposite ethical
decisions. This conflict cannot always be solved by balancing,
because rights are seen as very different kinds of things than
consequences. This is where protective responsibility comes
into play, as a second order consideration which defines that
the most important consideration must be that the patient is
not harmed. But apart from playing the role of a second order
consideration, protective responsibility also doubles as a virtue,
a way of contemplating and resolving ethical conflicts which
is possessed by the good professional and has strong similarities to Aristotle's concept of practical reasoning [80]. Protective
responsibility can thus be conceptualised as the source of both

respect and relationships, and of the more specific ethical considerations.

When the conflict occurs, and when the professional has decided that the harm is sufficiently significant to override the patient's wishes, various measures may be taken to 'persuade' the patient to do the right thing. Information can be given selectively, the patient can be 'threatened', or a decision may simply be imposed.

The patient in the centre

When the patient is fully competent, the role of relatives in the decision-making process is limited. When the patient's decision-making competence diminishes, the role of the relatives increases. But the treatment choices they propose are always evaluated carefully by the professional before they are carried out, and they are much more likely to be rejected than choices coming from the patient:

> R: *If we are talking about patients who are fully competent, then it is perfectly clear that you have to say that it must be the patient's own problem, and depend upon how much he trusts them, they have no right to interfere. But there can be situations where if, for instance, we have an older patient where a daughter calls about her mother, who may be poorly, and where the daughter wants some things done, and where I may talk a little with the daughter, and listen to what she is saying. And then we are together in saying these things to the mother, but there are situations where it is difficult to say exactly the same. But if I can see that the purpose is to get better conditions for the mother, then I will ease my duty of confidentiality a little with regard to the daughter, because the consideration of the patient's welfare weighs heavier on the scale.*
>
> I: *So it is the motive of the family which is —?*
>
> R: *Yes, it will probably be their motive and a judgement of how they are. I am very reluctant to do it on the phone. I ask them to come here and talk about it.* (DGM)

This process illustrates that the patient is the absolute centre of ethical decision-making, and although what is best for the family and what is best for society can be identified as individual ethical considerations in the arguments of some health care professionals, they always play a subsidiary role:

> It was a patient we had on the ward, a 70-year old man who had had a [...] stroke and who subsequently had epilepsy that was difficult to control. We could not control the seizures, that was his most important problem when we got him from {...} that his wife found it difficult to accept his seizures, and he had been in and out of {...} department of medicine, department of neurology, and was then sent home when the seizure was over, and they did not understand the wife, and were not very good at giving her support. Then he came to us. It quickly became clear that apart from the epilepsy he also had progressive dementia, and his somatic state also deteriorated. We treated his epilepsy, for some time very actively with diazepam, and he became almost comatose and was given intravenous fluids. He developed pneumonia, and one of the problems is that we felt that it was our treatment which made him almost comatose, but at the same time his wife came with a living will, or she came with a copy of the paper he, she had got from the register. So we knew that he had signed a statement that he did not want to be treated. And she was angry or upset that I had started fluids and penicillin for his pneumonia. We talked it over, and well, it was started, but know we knew something about it. [...] We had not removed all his seizures, but almost, and once in a while he was awake, and one day, just as I had talked with the nurse about what we could do, should we place a nasogastric tube, because he was on the list for nursing-home placement, but he could not go, and what was really supposed to happen. The same afternoon, and this is kind of funny, he was very lucid, and the nurse says to him 'What do you want? Should we give you fluids, should we give you a nasogastric tube?' − 'Well, if you don't I am going to die, and that I don't want.' Well, there we were with his living will and his present statement. At the same time we had many discussions with his wife, and one of the problems was that she treated him terribly. We had been on a visit to his home and she had been sitting with her back turned to him and talked about him as 'it'. So we had the feeling that if we followed the living will we were playing her game. But we still had the living will. [...] There were many problems involved, but in a way he solved it by saying 'Yes, I would like some food'. (DSF)

In some cases, professionals even feel a strong duty to protect patients against their families. This can happen when the decision-making capacity of the patient is permanently impaired, and the family demands specific treatment decisions which the professional judges as deleterious to the patient (this can be both too much or too little treatment):

> *There are times where it is so gross that you almost believe that the family stands to inherit money, it should be over with quickly, and at other times you know that there is nothing to inherit, but they have the same attitude anyway. I think that it is part of our job to explain to them why we do the things we do. It does not depend on the family. It is primarily the person we have in our care, and towards whom we have responsibility.* (DSM)

> *If I have to mention something which could point in the other direction, then it would be if you judge that this is not in the terminal phase. If you have the feeling that the 'demand' is put forward by the relatives, now you have to do it, she cannot take any more, and she has talked about it so many times, that kind of statement. If we have the feeling that it is the family's best interest you are asked to look after, and not the patient's, then it counts against starting, unless of course other factors are also present. I think that these are the two main reasons. That the patient is not terminal, and a less legitimate demand from the family.* (DSM)

Protective responsibility and ethical theory

In ethical theory protective responsibility as a basic concept has connections with the philosophy of the two German-Jewish philosophers Martin Buber and Hans Jonas [81, 71]. By tracing the similarities and differences between the concepts used by Buber and Jonas and protective responsibility it will be possible to get a better understanding of the content and limit of protective responsibility.

Through the aspects of respect and relationship, protective responsibility connects with Martin Buber's thought about the two kinds of relationship I can have with another being – the I–Thou relationship and the I–It relationship [81]. In the I–Thou relationship I meet the other being on a mutual basis, whereas in the I–It relationship the other being is reduced to a bundle of attributes, to a thing. Buber describes it in the following way:

I perceive something. I am sensible of something. I imagine something. I will something. I feel something. I think something. The life of human beings does not consist of all this and the like alone. This and the like together establish the realm of *It*.

But the realm of Thou has a different basis.

When *Thou* is spoken, the speaker has no thing for his object. For where there is a thing there is another thing. Every *It* is bounded by others; *It* exists only through being bounded by others. But when *Thou* is spoken, there is no thing. *Thou* has no bounds.

When *Thou* is spoken, the speaker has no *thing*; he has indeed nothing. But he takes his stand in relation. [81, p. 16–7, emphasis in original]

If I face a human being as my *Thou*, and say the primary words *I–Thou* to him, he is not a thing among things, and does not consist of things. [81, p. 21, emphasis in original]

Buber argues for an ethic that is dialogical, and against the attitude towards other people which disregards them as people and only sees them as things, collections of attributes, objects to be acted upon. His normative framework is therefore very pertinent to normative bioethics. Contrasting the I–Thou relationship with protective responsibility is also instructive because it sheds further light on the degree of personal involvement in protective responsibility.

The I–Thou relationship, as Buber describes it, is only established when the I (the person) reaches out, lets go of some of her or his defences, and leaves her or himself open to commune with the other. Establishing the I–Thou relationship requires effort, whereas the I–It relationship is always already given.

The relationship between professional and patient that is necessary to discharge protective responsibility in a suitable manner is different. On one level it is important never to let the patient be a mere thing, an It, but too close a relationship with the patient may also influence decisions and actions adversely. The old and venerable rule that physicians should not treat members of their own family is based partly on this duality in the importance of a close relationship. It is also fairly obvious that the effective performance of some medical interventions requiring brute force — for example, cardio-pulmonary resuscitation — is easier if the relationship with the patient and the recognition that the patient is a human person — can be bracketed during the procedure. We resuscitate because the patient is a person, but during the resuscitation we treat the patient as a thing. What we have, therefore, is a basic tension in protective responsibility. Protective responsibility requires a relationship with the patient, it should generate respect for the patient as a human being, but at the same time the professional has to be able to step back to assess what protection really amounts to in the present situation.

Protective responsibility connects with the ethics of Hans Jonas in another way. Jonas is interested in the increased power to alter the distant future which modern technology gives to humans. He argues that only an ethics of responsibility can handle this situation effectively, and only when it is coupled with a 'heuristic of fear' (that is, the methodological prescription that if you are presented with the promise of great benefit, and an equally likely risk of catastrophe, you should base your deliberations on the risk of catastrophe) [71].

As part of his theory Jonas develops an account of responsibility which states:

> The first and most general condition of responsibility is causal power, that is, that acting makes an impact on the world; the second, that such acting is under the agent's control; under these necessary conditions, there can be 'responsibility', but in two widely differing senses: (*a*) responsibility as being accountable 'for' one's deeds, whatever they are; and (*b*) responsibility 'for' particular objects that commits an agent to particular deeds concerning them. [71, p. 90]

Jonas argues that the second kind of responsibility has been underdeveloped in moral theory, but that it is this kind of responsibility that is most important. Although responsibility for one's acts is something every moral agent must shoulder, responsibility for others is the active force in Jonas's ethics. It is evident that this second kind of responsibility has close connections to the account of protective responsibility that has been extracted from the interviews in the present study.

Jonas further develops his account by contrasting two kinds of constant responsibility – parenting and statesmanship – where the former is seen as based in nature, and the latter as based in a self-chosen supererogatory act. What distinguishes parental and statesmen's responsibility from that of a physician is that on Jonas's view the responsibility of the physician is restricted in time and does not encompass the whole person:

> [T]he responsibility of the physician, begun with the therapeutic relationship, encompasses the curing, relief of suffering, and prolonging the life of the patient. All his other weal and woe lies outside its scope, and the 'worth' of the existence benefited or saved is none of its business. Total responsibility, however, must continually ask: 'What comes after that? Where will it lead?' and at the same time, 'What preceded it? How does what is happening now fit into the overall becoming of this existence?' [71, p. 106]

It seems to me that Jonas slightly underestimates the responsibility that health care professionals have to take on, and, at the very least, he definitely underestimates the responsibility they actually do take on.

The analysis of protective responsibility showed that health care professionals do primarily feel responsible for protecting the patient from evil (the bad effects caused by disease, etc.), and that they thereby see their responsibility as restricted in scope at any given time (that is, they are not responsible for making the patient happy). The responsibility they accept is not, however, restricted temporally in the way Jonas suggests. In many cases some of the questions asked are exactly – 'What comes after that? Where will it lead?' It is true that the possibility to have a direct affect ends when the patient leaves hospital or when the treatment and care is otherwise finished, and that the possibility to discharge a responsibility for the patient thereby diminishes. But this is in one sense not different from Jonas's own analysis of the final stage of parental responsibility, when the child has reached adulthood. Independent adulthood is (or should be) the goal of parenting, and parental responsibility as an ongoing activity ends when this goal is reached. But many of the actions taken during the upbringing of the child, and many of the reasons behind these actions,

point further on in time than the moment of attaining adulthood.

In the same way, the actions and considerations of health
care professionals do not only take into account the short
period of time between the admission and discharge of the
patient. Many of them are directed towards enabling the
patient to act in certain ways long after the treatment period
is over. Protective responsibility is, in this sense, extended in
time far beyond the identifiable treatment period.

Protective responsibility and power

The concept of protective responsibility is also connected to
Howard Brody's analysis of the three kinds of power that
health care professionals possess [82]. In *The Healer's Power*
Brody distinguishes between Aesculapian power, charismatic
power, and social power. Aesculapian power is what professionals possess because of their knowledge about disease, illness, and therapeutic options. Charismatic power is derived
from the professional's personality and position in the social
stratification. And social power is given to the professional
through recognised social mechanisms (e.g., permission to do
certain acts which are normally prohibited, permission to issue
certain documents with legal effects, etc.). Brody argues that
because health care professionals, and especially doctors, have
these powers, they also have specific responsibilities.

With regard to the ethical exercise of power, Brody points
out that it must be aimed at the right goal, shared with the
patient as far as possible, and owned or recognised by the professional (that is, that the use of power is not covert). Further,
he argues that it is not sufficient to focus exclusively on the
acts performed by the professional (the use of power); a full
ethical analysis must also include the dispositions or virtues
that a person must possess to recognise when and how to use
power. He identifies the virtue of compassion as the most
important, leading to a responsible use of power:

> We are now in a position to see why the virtue of compassion is
> integrally linked to the ethical use of power in the
> physician–patient relationship. Surely, being with the sufferer and

helping him find his own story to attach meaning to his experience is a prime example of shared power. Few things that the physician can do have the capacity to empower the patient to a similar degree. Disease may threaten bodily function and bodily integrity; suffering threatens one's connections with humanity and one's ability to make sense of one's own life. If the physician attends only to disease and ignores suffering, he may cure but still fail to heal …
. To be compassionate in response to the suffering of the patient is therefore one of the most powerful things a physician can do; but this is possible only to the extent that the physician is willing to adopt a position of relative powerlessness, to acknowledge that the patient's suffering has incredible power over him and that he cannot remain unchanged in the face of it.

…

It may be largely out of this dual sense of power and humility that the physician's virtue and character can help insure that power is used responsibly and its abuses are avoided. Owned, aimed, and shared power each arise naturally from this dual sense of power and humility engendered by the virtue of compassion. [82, p. 259–60]

Brody's argument aims at uncovering what kind of virtues and dispositions professionals *ought* to have. It is therefore not surprising that he ends up with a description of the virtue he calls compassion, which is only partially congruent with the concept of protective responsibility found here in a descriptive study. Direct naming of power is rare in the interviews in the present study, but there is clear recognition that what health care professionals do may profoundly change the lives of other people. This recognition forms the basis for protective responsibility, which, under an unfriendly interpretation, is a truncation of Brody's virtue of compassion, but which under a more friendly interpretation, can be seen to be a realistic and appropriate adaptation of his ideal.

It could be claimed that the lack of explicit power-talk in the interviews signifies false-consciousness on the part of the professionals interviewed. They have power, but they do not own up to it, therefore they display false-consciousness. On a Marxist analysis this would be the inevitable conclusion. On the other side it could be claimed that although the word 'power' is rarely used, other words and phrases like 'influence', 'authority', 'status', and 'important decision' occur frequently. Power-talk is present, but in a slightly different form. In this context it is interesting to note that perceived powerlessness has been found to correlate with ethical decision-making. One study has found that the more powerless a nurse feels, the greater is the risk that he or she makes inappropriate ethical decisions [21]. If this is true, power may be necessary for good ethical decisions.

Where does ethics come from?

Other aspects of the core concept of protective responsibility can be illuminated by looking at the respondents' theories about how ethical attitudes are created. What is it that gives one person high ethical standards, and turns others into more dubious characters? By looking at this question it is possible to find out more about whether protective responsibility is seen as a moral principle or as a moral virtue.

In the material analysed there is an interesting dichotomy between the belief that ethical standards are mainly a question of personality, and a belief that they can be raised by discussion and education. These two beliefs are held simultaneously by many respondents, and they seem, on the face of it, to be inconsistent.

Ethics as a personality trait

If we look at the belief that ethical standards are mainly a question of personality, we see that it has two distinct parts. The first is the belief as it has already been stated, and the second is the belief that a person's personality is fixed at an early stage of development and is a product of her or his upbringing:

> When you say doctors, it implies postgraduate and I think that is too late. I don't think you can, I would almost say, correct the faults in the crystal at that time. And I actually think that it is something which begins with toilet training. It is something we ourselves begin very early in the way we bring up our children, and our years in

school are also filled with ethical considerations. Discussions about good and bad. So I think that if you have been through all of this and have become a medical doctor without being deeply involved in these discussions and considerations, then I don't think it is something you can repair in order to function as a doctor. And again, it begins when you are a child observing the attitudes and actions of your parents, whether there is agreement between what they say, and what they do. So it is something which has to start early on, and, to put it very simplistically, I think that if you have begun very early, and if you come from a background where these things have been discussed, then you are going to be a better doctor. It is my firm opinion that if it is something which you have never considered, and have put aside and said 'it is not my problem', then it is very unfortunate. (DSM)

I think, as I said before, that basically it is the way you view other people that decides how you think. You cannot, there are some things, you cannot change attitudes toward life, it is at least very difficult. (DIM)

At the limit, this set of beliefs entails that high ethical standards are a stable personality trait (virtue?) which is acquired in childhood, and which it is very difficult to change. External pressure may force the unethical person to conform and behave in acceptable ways, but it does not change her or his ethical standards. What we should do in order to get ethical health care professionals is to select carefully among those wanting to enter professional training.

That ethical standards are really seen as a stable personality trait is further supported by the account the respondents give about the effects of hierarchical positions on ethical reasoning. Almost without exception these accounts involve the claim that a person's ethical standards are constant – only the vantage point, the level of information, and the type of ethical problems that have to be considered, change:

The thing which changes when you move upward in the hierarchy is that you get possibilities to see the issues in a broader context, and you get a different background for your judgements than you have at other levels in the hierarchy, but there is no change in morality. It is a change of the basis for the decisions, which can be somewhat different, and lead to somewhat different actions. The morality itself is not changed. (DSM)

The only kind of people who are believed possibly to lose their morality by moving upward in the hierarchy are those who move from a position with actual clinical contact with the patients to a purely administrative position. Two respondents mention that, in their experience, such a move may cause some people to lose their ethical standards.

The effects of education

The belief that education can help has two forms, which differ in the kind of 'education' that is seen as effective. For some, the effective kind of education is the good example given by superiors in word and deed, whereas others believe that direct education in the form of courses or educational discussions can be fruitful:

> I think it is a teaching process. For myself it has at least been the contact with various chiefs through the years, where you have learnt about their attitudes and their way of behaving, and about whether they have thought about working according to these principles, that is what I have adopted for myself. (DSM)

> I should like to advocate a return of the old introductory philosophy course, maybe in a medical version, but I do not think, that you can look at medical ethics without a philosophical basis. My proposal would be to reintroduce the introductory philosophy course, maybe with some reference to medical interests; and I think it had a manageable size back then, so I think it can be done. (DSM)

But even though there is this difference in the assessment of different kinds of education, almost all respondents believe that education in ethics is a good thing which can help people to make better ethical decisions.

Personality or education?

Can these two seemingly inconsistent beliefs about the genesis and mutability of a person's ethical standards be united in any way? For the respondents themselves there is no problem:

> I am totally convinced, that in those situations where it goes wrong, it is because of the personality of the individual employee. And the personality is also influenced by the knowledge of the individual employee, because when we discuss things I experience that they are

all, that they all learn very easily. Yes, as I said, I think the staff is very good at learning these things, but you have an attitude based on what you have learned before, and it is obvious that there are many things that can be learned, and thank God for that. (NSM)

On a theoretical level it is more difficult to reconcile the two points of view, but perhaps the assertion of compatibility just quoted gives a hint as to how a reconciliation may be accomplished after all. This is perhaps best shown if we begin with the concept of 'protective responsibility' again.

What follows with respect to singular ethical decisions, and more general ethical rules such as 'do not lie to patients', if we accept that protective responsibility is a core notion in the system of ethical thought used by health care professionals? It follows that any decision or rule must be appropriately connected to the core concept, but it does not follow that a person having the system of ethical thought based on this core concept also has the full set of rules that the system can contain. Or, to put it differently, there may be rules derivable from the system which the person has not yet seen or realised. Conversely, a person may hold rules which on reflection can be shown to be incompatible with the core of the ethical system. As discussed above in the section about ethical perception, ethical decision-making may in some instances become routinised (almost habitual), and this may have both good and bad effects.

If a person lacks rules that are derivable from, or holds rules which are really incompatible with, the ethical system, education can make a difference. The discrepancies can be pointed out, and the person may be able to change her or his ideas about the ethically correct thing to do in specific situations. What education does, on this conception, is not so much change the ethics of the person; the main gain is achieved by clarification and conceptualisation of the ethics which the person already possesses, with protective responsibility as a stable reference point.

But this does not solve the problem of the unethical person, who is presumably characterised either by not having a system of ethics (that is, being amoral), or by having a system that does not contain anything like protective responsibility (he or she may, for instance, be an ethical egoist). The respondents do not have any answer to how such people might be 'improved', except that their actions must be kept within ethical bounds, either by peer pressure, or by the other coercive measures available in the organisation (see Chapter 5).

The dichotomy between personality and education can therefore not be totally dissolved. Health care professionals believe that there are people whose personality structures are such that they are 'beyond redemption', and beyond the reach of any educational attempts. There are, however, only a few such people, and for the great majority education can play a role.

> The reason why I don't just answer yes or no is that we have all met people of whom you say that even if they were only 10 years of age it would be too late to change anything, and on the other hand, you now and again meet people who are in their late 60s or even older, and who begin to reflect on various topics and say, God, here we have really acted wrongly or differently or why have I not thought about this before. If you are receptive to those kinds of things, then you can enjoy it and that is the reason why we should keep on, even if we know that there is a minority where you can scream and shout and try to educate and send them on courses or whatever without any effect at all, but that shouldn't keep you from trying. (DSM)

Problematisation of the personality explanation

There is reason to believe that the content of the ethical reasoning of health care professionals differs from that of 'ordinary people', and an explanation of the ethical standard of health care professionals in terms of stable personality traits or character developed in childhood or adolescence can therefore be problematic. How can the differences be explained if a person's ethical standards and ethical reasoning are determined before he or she chooses a career in health care?

Self-selection of persons with high ethical standards to health care occupations is a possible explanation, but it is not reasonable to assume that it is the only explanation (e.g., a career in medicine can also be chosen for its social status and prestige).

Another possible explanation would parallel that given for the importance of education. If we assume that people's basic ethical frameworks are settled during their upbringing, then it will presumably still be the case that there is some flexibility within those frameworks. In adult life each occupation gives rise to a distinct set of ethical problems (e.g., policemen, lawyers, teachers, and nurses all encounter ethical problems but the problems are not the same), and the ethical considerations that are pertinent to the solution of these problems are therefore likely gradually to assume a more prominent place in the ethical framework. According to this explanation, differences between different occupational groups are explained by their differential exposure to ethical problems, and by the concomitant selection of those ethical considerations that are most useful in a given occupation. This would, for instance, mean that although protective responsibility is probably present in the ethical framework of 'ordinary people', its prominent role in the ethical framework of health care professionals is due to its 'usefulness' in resolving their specific ethical problems. This explanation is, in a sense, only a version of Aristotle's explanation of the development of prudence:

> There is also confirmation of what we have said in the fact that although the young develop ability in geometry and mathematics and become wise in such matters, they are not thought to develop prudence. The reason for this is that prudence also involves knowledge of particular facts, which become known from experience; and a young man is not experienced, because experience takes some time to acquire' *(EN 1142a12–16)* [80, pp. 214–15]

Ethics education – when and how?

Ethics education is seen as effective and worthwhile for the great majority of health care professionals, but when should it take place, and how should it be done?

The first question is easy to answer. Ethics education should not, in the view of the respondents, be confined to one separate segment of professional life, but should have a place in both undergraduate and postgraduate training, and as continuing education courses for the fully educated professional. Apart from formal courses, it should also be integrated in the day-to-day function of hospital departments.

The second question is more difficult to answer, because the respondents identify a significant interaction between practical experience of problem situations and the value of formal education. Ethical theory may be a good thing to learn, but it is sterile if it cannot be connected to the experience of the students.

Based on this general view many different suggestions are made, ranging from a reintroduction of the old apprenticeship-like relationship between senior and junior professionals, through targeted case conferences, to more formalised ethics courses with an emphasis on the ethical problems of health care professionals. What is needed is not just 'knowledge' but 'living knowledge', which is applicable in daily work:

> *You should teach them what ethics is. I think that many − if you asked my colleagues, what ethics is and would you like to be taught about it − they would probably not know what content, I am not quite certain either about what content such teaching should have, but it is precisely to get some concepts elaborated and contrasted against each other. I think that for many of us ethics is something which deals with specific things, and we could probably benefit from being told that it is not just something about sitting in a small room studying like the philosopher, that it is actually about something concrete, that it deals concretely with our world. And what norms and such you adopt is not, according to my opinion, what ethical education should result in. But you should present the norms, systematise them, and make it into something specific, something living for us. I think that would be good. It also makes it easier when we get a concept, some words to put on some issues we sometimes encounter without knowing what to call them. Ethics teaching could help us here.* (DSF)

This quote again exemplifies that ethics education is seen as a help to organise and conceptualise an ethic which is in some sense already present.

A complete model of ethical reasoning

The ethical reasoning process elucidated in this chapter can be summarised in two figures. The first of these (Figure 4.2) shows the interrelationship between the components of the ethical framework involved in the reasoning stages of the process.

Figure 4.2 Interrelationships in the clinical framework

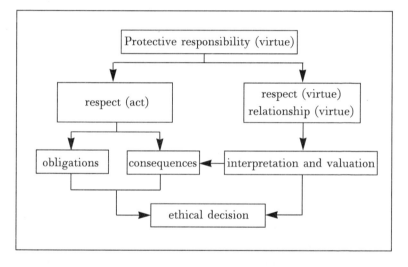

The second figure (Figure 4.3) tries to show the whole process from perception of an ethical problem to implementation of a solution. As mentioned above, a strictly linear model is not able to explain the ethical decision-making process of the health care professionals studied here. First, the process takes place within three overlapping 'spaces'; an ethical space delimited by the ethical framework, a personal space defined by personal experiences and character, and an organisational space delimited by the structure, process, and culture of the hospital, etc. (see Chapter 5). Factors in these spaces influence all parts of the decision-making process. In the model shown

Figure 4.3 The ethical decision-making process

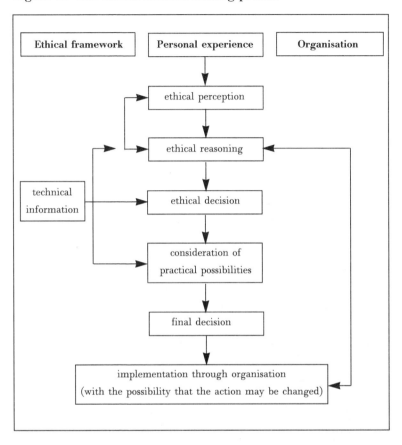

here there should, therefore, have been arrows indicating influence from the three frames to all parts of the process. Second there are several steps where information is injected into the decision-making process, and two feedback loops, between ethical perception and ethical reasoning and between ethical reasoning and implementation of a decision.

Perspectives from health care ethics

The overall structure of the model of ethical decision-making is rather similar to the model in Ajzen's theory of planned behaviour, in which behaviour is seen as explained by intentions that are shaped by perceived control, social norms, and attitudes towards the behaviour [83]. If the behaviour also includes an ethical component, a further element of moral obligation can be incorporated [84]. In a study of nurses' willingness to report other professionals who delivered suboptimal care, Randall and Gibson found that Ajzen's theory could explain 'a significant amount of the variation in the intent to report a colleague' [85, p. 111].

In the literature on ethical perception and reasoning there are otherwise only a few studies similar to this present one. Omery used qualitative methods to study the ethical reasoning of ten American intensive care nurses [86]. Lützén used observation, and combined grounded theory and phenomenological methods to study ethical aspects of psychiatric nursing. Based on this research she conducted a grounded theory study of the moral sensitivity of fourteen Swedish psychiatric nurses, and developed a moral sensitivity scale [87]. Udén *et al.* used narrative theory to analyse forty-three stories about ethically difficult care situations obtained in interviews with twenty-three nurses and nine physicians in Norway [88]. I have not been able to find any other studies using qualitative methods to investigate the ethical reasoning of physicians.

When the findings of the present study are compared to the findings in Omery's, Lützén's and Udén's studies, both similarities and differences can be found. Omery first identifies two different kinds of moral reasoner, whom she calls accommodating and sovereign. Accommodating reasoners 'adjusted, adapted, or reconciled their moral judgments to conform with the perceived norm of the dominant group', whereas sovereign reasoners 'based their moral judgments on self-chosen moral principles which were valued by that individual' [86, p. 77]. She then identifies the principles used by these reasoners. Both types of reasoners use the principles of honesty and responsibility. The sovereign reasoners also use care, advocacy, autonomy, respect, fairness, quality of life, and (no) intent to harm; and the accommodating reasoners use avoidance, paternalism, reciprocity, professional protectionalism, legalism, and consensus [86, p.79].

I only discovered Omery's study after the analysis process of the present study was completed. I therefore performed a quick re-analysis focusing only on the question of whether or not her distinction between accommodating and sovereign reasoners could be applied. This re-analysis showed that no respondents in the present study could unequivocally be labelled as accommodating reasoners. A few of the physicians and one nurse had strong accommodating features in their ethical reasoning, but these were always mixed with sovereign features. When I compare my findings with Omery's I therefore confine myself to her account of the moral reasoning of sovereign reasoners.

It is interesting that one of the two most important principles she identified by Omery is responsibility. Her description of the principle is as follows:

> Sovereign reasoners described themselves as being responsible to the patients. In any moral situation, sovereign reasoners would describe themselves as accountable to the patient to provide optimal and competent nursing care. These reasoners consistently expanded the principle of responsibility to include themselves. That is, in any moral dilemma, they had an obligation to be accountable to themselves for their moral judgment and action. As one stated:
>
> > My responsibility would be to myself and to the client. This is a catalyst and enzyme situation. One doesn't go without the other for optimal care and concern. [86, p. 82]

What mainly distinguishes Omery's responsibility from protective responsibility as described in this study is, first, that protective responsibility is narrower in the sense that it places priority on protection from harm, and second, that protective responsibility can best be understood as a virtue, and not as a principle.

Omery also identifies the mediating external factors which influence ethical reasoning and finds that the situation, legal constraints, and the nurse–physician relationship are the three major mediating factors [86, p. 92]. Within the situation she

further identifies three essential aspects; the objective facts, the
specific individuals involved, and the interpersonal dynamics
[86, p. 93]. In this area there is general agreement between her
findings and the findings in the present study about the factors which influence perception of ethical problems. The only
major discrepancy is that legal considerations play a much
larger role in America than in Denmark, which can easily be
explained by the very large difference in the amount of medical litigation in the two countries.

In Lützén's two qualitative studies a number of concepts
are developed. The two main ones that she derives from the
observation study are moral sensing and ideological conflict,
where moral sensing is defined as: 'a type of *sensitivity* to the
moral meaning of actions taken in a situation where one
person is dependent on another' [87, p. 27, emphasis in origi-
nal]. In her interview study she identifies three further concepts, which can be seen as extensions and clarifications of the
moral sense concept. These are 'structuring moral meaning' as
the core concept, and 'expressing benevolence' and 'modifying
autonomy' as subsidiary concepts. She defines them in the following way:

> 'Structuring moral meaning' identifies a spontaneous process aimed
> at solving moral conflict. This process was prior to action and
> included integrating all known aspects of the context and past
> experiences in order to make sense of a new and unique situation.
> For the nurses, 'Structuring moral meaning' begins when the nurse
> attempts to weave the fragments of the situation into a whole. This
> entails perceiving the patient's vulnerability in relationship to her
> own actions. [87, p. 30]

> The subsidiary concept, 'expressing benevolence', the desire to do
> 'good' ..., describes the motivating factor, justifying making deci-
> sions for the patient in each situation. This involves responding to
> the patient's vulnerability which in these accounts, meant taking a
> risk by placing the professional role in jeopardy if 'wrong' action
> was taken. [87, pp. 30–1]

> Modifying autonomy', is defined as adjusting the meaning of self-
> choice to suit the perceived needs of the patient. [87, p. 31]

Again, there are both similarities and differences in comparison with the findings in the present study. The emphasis on the vulnerability of the patient as a significant factor in moral decision-making matches the concept of protective responsibility that I have described as the core concept in moral reasoning; the emphasis on the necessity to structure moral meaning by taking account of the context of each new situation matches my description of the process of ethical perception, and modifying autonomy, although not an independent concept in my analysis, does figure in the development of protective responsibility. The main difference at the concept level concerns Lützén's concept 'expressing benevolence'. In protective responsibility a similar idea is integrated, but not as a general benevolence, only as a benevolence aimed at protecting the patient from harm.

The other main difference is the way in which the whole situation of moral decision-making is conceptualised, where I try to maintain a sharper distinction between the steps of ethical perception and ethical decision-making than Lützén. If this difference is taken into account, the two sets of concept developed here and by Lützén look very similar.

The work by Udén et al. is not as directly relevant to the present study as the two others discussed above, because it is not as directly focused on ethical reasoning, but it does identify a number of interesting differences between the stories told by nurses and the stories told by physicians. Their findings are summarised as themes in Table 4.4 [modified from 88, p. 1031]. Whether these themes represent differences in ethical considerations, in ethical perception, or in a more general perspective on professional life is difficult to establish from the article describing the study. It is also hard to see what definition of paternalism the authors have used, and it is therefore not easy to discuss whether there is any major discrepancy between their findings and the findings in the present study.

No directly comparable Danish studies can be found. In a study of wishes for terminal care in nursing homes, Moe found that nurses and assistant nurses utilised the concepts of good and bad quality of life, conscience and responsibility, and the resident's wishes in explaining hypothetical decisions about whether or not to transfer the patient to hospital or treat actively in other ways [89]. Among these considerations, quality of life seemed the most important. It is difficult to compare Moe's finding to the present study because the main focus of his research was not ethical reasoning, and because he only studied arguments concerning one specific set of decisions. Two surveys of samples of the Danish general population in 1981 and 1990 indicate that most people have what the authors label as a high public morality, and that the proportion having this high public morality is not changing very much. The public morality measure incorporates attitudes toward actions performed as a public official, and attitudes towards private actions with a significant public component [90]. This study is not directly relevant to the analysis of ethical reasoning of professionals, but it describes the general environment within which their reasoning occurs.

Table 4.4   Themes occurring in nurses' and physicians' stories

Nurses' stories	Physicians' stories
retrospectively	prospectively
health and daily life	disease
experimental knowledge	scientific knowledge
closeness to the patient	distance
patient autonomy	paternalism
quality of life	preserving life
pessimism	optimism
death with dignity	survival
powerlessness	power
being together with colleagues	being isolated as an individual

Nurses, doctors and caring

The literature on nursing ethics, and parts of the literature on moral reasoning (see Chapter 1) posit quite sharp distinctions between nursing ethics and medical ethics, and between the moral reasoning of women and men. In the analysis of the present data I therefore tried to be open to these differences, but apart from the fact that, for nurses, relationships with patients are more important than they are for doctors, no differences were found in the individual ethical considerations or in the overall structure of the ethical framework. Likewise, the concept of care was kept in mind in the analysis phase, but was not found to be a core concept in the moral reasoning of the group of nurses or the group of women in this study.

Given the non-random nature of the sample in the present study, and the mode of analysis, it is not possible to give any statistical estimates of how accurate these findings are in a numerical sense, but the same is true of a number of the studies in the literature reporting significant differences. These findings differ from a substantial number of theoretical and empirical studies of the ethical reasoning of doctors and nurses. A listing and detailed discussion of all these studies would be beside the point here. Possible explanations of the contradictory findings range from the almost inevitable *ad hominem* that the present study was performed by a male doctor, and that the result was therefore predictable, to more serious possibilities.

Many of the empirical studies identifying care as a significant factor in the moral reasoning of nurses have been conducted in the USA, and the cultural differences in gender and nursing socialisation may, at least partly, explain the apparent differences in moral reasoning. Another possible explanation may be that the present study was not confined to looking at ethical principles. If other types of ethical concepts are brought in (virtues, dispositions) the opposition between an attitude of care and the principle of justice may be seen to occur within a larger framework, where none of these two considerations is the major consideration. In the present study care could be seen as 'parcelled out' as parts of protective responsibility and relationship.

Relations to moral philosophy

The ethical framework described here contains elements from

consequentialism, deontological ethics, and virtue theory, but does not fit neatly into any of these three categories, although it is most closely related to virtue theory. In the following paragraphs I shall briefly review the connections with each of the three classical types of theory, and then move on to some of the more modern attempts to construct an integrated model of medical ethics, with special emphasis on models trying to take account of virtue ethics.

In comparison with standard consequentialism two things are worth noting. The first of these is that within the present framework consequences matter, but good consequences are not the only form of ethical consideration that is seen as valid or important. Rights, obligations, and virtues also play a role. The respondents would therefore probably endorse the critique of consequentialism put forward by, for instance, Williams and Dancy, who both claim that consequentialist theory simply misses a lot of what is morally important [91, 92].

The second is that the ethical framework described here is not impartial in any strong sense (the interests of all are not given equal weight), but it is weakly impartial in the sense that the interests of all those occupying the same specific position or role (e.g., as patient, relative, professional, etc.) are given equal consideration and weight in the deliberation.

Wulff *et al.* describe 'patient-orientated utilitarianism' as a possible ethical position that health care professionals could adopt in their clinical work [93]. In other words, a utilitarian mode of reasoning where the thing to be maximised is the utility for the patient (that is,. the individual patient whose problems I am currently contemplating) [93]. This theoretical position is congruent with the consequentialist part of the framework described here, but it does not admit any room for rights, duties, respect, or relationship.

The framework also has connections to deontological ethics. A number of rights and obligations are recognised, and some of these fit nicely with the traditional lists of dos and don'ts. Even so, the importance given to the patients' best interests makes it impossible to claim that it is a deontological framework. If it was seen as such there would also be the prob-

lem that none of the rights and obligations are absolute and
there are no strict priority rules. There is no way within the
rights and duties part of the framework to resolve conflict
between rights. This resolution comes from other parts of the
framework.

Finally, there are connections to traditional virtue theory.
The framework contains at least three elements that are best
conceptualised as virtues held by the good professional – that
is, the core concept of protective responsibility and the concepts
of respect and relationship. A characteristic of classical virtue
theory is that there is no formulaic method of reaching the
correct decision in ethical problems, and this is also an important component of the ethics of health care professionals. The
framework is also connected to virtue theory through the
emphasis put on the importance of context in ethical deliberation. The recognition of the concreteness of each situation is
an important part of Aristotelian practical reasoning, as Nussbaum notes:

> Being responsibly committed to the world of value before her, the
> perceiving agent can be counted on to investigate and scrutinize the
> nature of each item and each situation, to respond to what is there
> before her with full sensitivity and imaginative vigor, not to fall
> short of what is there to be seen and felt because of evasiveness,
> scientific abstractness, or a love of simplification. The Aristotelian
> agent is a person whom we could trust to describe a complex situ-
> ation with full concreteness of detail and emotional shading, miss-
> ing nothing of practical relevance. [94, p. 84]

Most health care professionals (as well as most other people)
fall short of this ideal, but this does not detract from the fact
that recognition of the relevant contextual features is seen as
extremely important.

In modern medical ethics all kinds of theoretical
approaches have been tried. In the following section I will confine myself to compare the framework identified here with
some of the medical ethics approaches which take virtue
theory seriously. Further comparison with mainstream consequentialist or deontological medical ethics would probably not
lead to any further illumination.

In *Theory and Practice in Medical Ethics* Graber and Thomasma describe, analyse, and criticise a number of different ways in which the relationship between ethical theory and clinical practice can be conceptualised [95]. They then present their own way of thinking, which partly builds on previous work by Thomasma and Pellegrino, who analysed medicine as a practice (an Aristotelian *techne*), and argued that certain moral ideals could be derived directly from the inherent values in the practice of medicine [96]. According to Graber and Thomasma:

> a unitary theory of clinical ethics must rely on the virtues of the interpreter(s) of the crisis situation and deontological guidelines for the conscience of the interpreter(s). In medicine those guidelines are provided by the moral nature of the enterprise itself, by the social and cultural mores, as well as by applications of more general ethical theory. Nonetheless it is the interpreter(s) who must do the applying, mediation, determination, validation, and origination not only about the decisions but also about the inductive and deductive products of which we spoke in earlier chapters. Just as in modern scientific theory the role of the observer has received critical attention, so too should it in medical ethics [95, p. 192]

Virtues are here seen as necessary in clinical ethics because case interpretation and application of principles are always done by specific people (the interpreters). If we do not have specific rules describing exactly how cases should be described and understood, and exactly how principles should be applied, the necessity of interpretation will also make virtues necessary in order to 'fill the gap' between situation and principles.

The authors then define their unitary theory in the following way: 'Certain conditions are present in this case such that the probability (x) exists that Value A will be judged more important than B by interpreters because the principle p' will more likely apply to the case than p" [95, p. 194]. This attempt at devising a unitary theory of clinical ethics has a structure that is very similar to that of the ethical reasoning of health care professionals identified in this study, where a set of virtues underlies both the identification and application of a set of values and principles. The virtues which Graber and Thomasma see as important are, however, the traditional list of physicians' virtues (benevolence, honesty etc.). This is a feature which recurs in many of the applications of virtue theory in medical ethics. Often, rather long lists of virtues are proposed without any attempt to prioritise or integrate them (e.g., Gorovitz's list of characteristics of the good physician comprises thirteen characteristics/virtues [97, pp. 192–3]).

In a framework where virtues rights and duties, and consequences are given a place, this proliferation of virtues is not necessary. There is, for instance, no need to posit a virtue of honesty if it is more appropriate to posit a duty to tell the truth. That the ethical framework of health care professionals only incorporates the three virtues of protective responsibility, respect, and relationship, is therefore not necessarily a defect in the framework, since it also recognises rights and consequences.

In a theory recognising the importance of virtues, rights, and consequences, there are at least three different ways in which virtues can be conceptualised. They can be seen as additional − that is, as belonging to a separate part of the theory dealing not with right action but, for instance, with blame and punishment. They can also be seen as mediating − that is, as important when principles are in conflict − and they will thus play no role in deciding on the content of principles, but only come into play if principles derived from elsewhere in the theory come into conflict. Finally, they can be seen as alternatives to rights and obligations, so that at least some principles become superfluous and are replaced by virtues; or it could be the case that principles were derived from the virtues. The ethical framework described here seems to assign to the virtues of protective responsibility, respect, and relationship a role which is both mediating and alternative.

I have already pointed out several times that protective responsibility is more restricted than benevolence or beneficence, because it is mainly concerned with protection from harm and not with general well-being or doing good. In this way protective responsibility is less demanding than benevolence and beneficence, because the problems concerning proper discharge of a duty to protect are less than those concerning a duty to do good. This assertion is perhaps not immediately obvious, but it can be supported by the following considerations.

It is a common-place observation that we can never fully discharge an impartial duty of beneficence. There is no way in which we can help all the people who are in need, and whom we theoretically should help. We may be able to benefit all, but we will never be able to benefit all to the extent they need it. And even if we restrict the scope of the duty to cover only the patients in one's care, there would probably always be some extra thing which could be done to benefit them. Beneficence must therefore be an imperfect duty. I have a duty to help people in need, but exactly who I am obligated to help is not specified in the duty itself.

Acts protecting from harm constitute a subclass of beneficent acts, but if the number of possible beneficent acts is infinite, the number of acts in any subclass can also be infinite, so there is no simple numerical argument showing that it is easier to discharge a duty to protect from harm. If there are no restrictions on the scope of the duty, the predictive time-scale, and the types of harm, the duty *is* probably undischargeable. If I have to take all harms into account no matter how far in the future they occur, and no matter whom they affect, there would be so many of them that my entire time would be spent avoiding them. If, however, the scope is restricted to the patients who are presently in my care, the type of harm is restricted to that which is causally connected to disease and illness, and the time-frame is restricted to, say, ten years, then the duty might be dischargeable (whether it is or not is to some extent an empirical question). A duty of beneficence would, even with the same restrictions, still be undischargeable because of the open-endedness of the possibility to do good.

That health care professionals incorporate protective responsibility in their ethical framework instead of benevolence may be seen as a prudent adaptation to the real world.

Problem areas in the professional ethical framework

When evaluated from the outside, the ethical framework held by health care professionals and analysed in this chapter contain two major problem areas; paternalism and justice.

Although protective responsibility is not the same as paternalism, and does not in itself warrant paternalistic action, it is evident that the step from protective responsibility to paternalism is very short. If 'doing what is best for the patient' is interpreted without adequate emphasis on the value and importance of autonomy, the distinction between protective responsibility and paternalism may disappear. In this context it is important to note that paternalism is not necessarily a bad thing, unless it is defined so as to exclude wanted paternalism (for example, in cases where the patient asks the health care professional to decide), and genuine paternalism (for example, in cases where the patient is really in a situation resembling that of a child because of various impediments to autonomous decision-making).

In the interviews conducted for this study it is clear that respect for autonomy plays a large role in ethical considerations, but that the right to autonomous decisions is not seen as an absolute right. If there is too large a discrepancy between what the patient wants and what is judged to be best for the patient, the latter may become the overriding consideration, and un-wanted paternalism may be the consequence. Within the ethical framework there is thus an unresolved tension between two understandings of what 'respecting the patient' amounts to ('respecting autonomy' or 'respecting best interest'). Although there is broad agreement in bioethics that paternalism is a bad thing, there is still disagreement about whether paternalism is *always* a bad thing. That the ethical framework described here leaves room for paternalism is not necessarily a sign that there is something fundamentally wrong in the framework, as long as the room left for it is small.

A model of the professional–patient relationship in which the professional is only an adviser and the patient is the sole decision-maker is unrealistic. It is impossible to distinguish

medical facts and value judgments in such a way that the professional can give the patient value-free information. Fully
implemented, an adviser or scientific model would also entail,
that the professional would not have to make any ethical decisions, or as Burke expresses it: 'The irony is that this model,
which champions the physician's scientific knowledge, would
leave him a moral illiterate' [98, p. 618]. Because value-free
information is a fiction the clinical practice of medicine and
nursing is inherently paternalistic to some extent, and an element of trust between patient and professional is necessary [99].

A residual worry could be that the consideration which
blocks paternalism in most cases – respecting autonomy – is
historically new in the ethical framework of health care professionals, and might therefore be a relatively weak consideration. The present analysis cannot support that worry. It also
seems to be the case that society in general is moving in the
direction of more emphasis on autonomy, and this should, all
other things being equal, lead to greater protection against
unwarranted paternalism.

The other problem area centres around justice considerations and the recognition of the possible social causes of a
patient's problems. Because the core components of the framework are concerned with the specific patient, there are problems in accommodating broader issues of justice.

Bioethics has in general been accused of looking too closely
at individual problem cases, and neglecting the larger social
issues which may create the individual problems [100]. This
critique is justified with regard to bioethics as such, and it also
seems justified when we look at the ethical framework of the
health care professionals in this study. The problems they see,
the considerations they apply, and the solutions they propose
are all centred on the individual patient. Any kind of social critique is only raised if unfavourable societal changes directly
impinge on the providing of health care (see the section 'Exit,
voice, obstruction, and loyalty' in Chapter 5).

The other aspect of this problem is reflected in public discussions about resource allocation in health care, where health
care professionals often claim that if they could just have more

money the need for explicit resource allocation would go away. This point of view is often linked to an assertion that at some point (never exactly specified) in the past, doctors did not take resources into account in their decisions, but decided solely on the basis of medical (technical) considerations. This is obviously a fiction, in the sense that doctors may well have believed and felt that they only took medical considerations into account, but that belief was based on an exaggeration of the decisiveness of technical considerations. Other factors have always played a role.

In the present material this attitude is exemplified in the responses to case 6, describing an elderly man with cancer of the prostate and bronchitis, who is admitted to hospital with an attack of bronchitis. In connection with an argument about whether a prior decision should be made not to offer respiratory support, one of the physicians offered the following remarks:

> But I don't think that you should ask the patients, whether they want to be treated for their next bout of pneumonia. I think that we have to take responsibility for the treatment, and we have to know whether it is futile or not futile. (DIF)

According to the information given in this case, the patient is not terminally ill, so a decision about futility cannot be a decision about technical futility. What we see, therefore, is a moral decision, or a resource allocation decision, disguised/redescribed as a technical decision about futility. We have some empirical evidence supporting the idea that futility is not a firm medical/technical criterion. In a study of American physicians Van McCrary *et al.* found that the cut-off point for the rate of success that physicians used to decide whether a treatment for a terminally ill patient was futile varied between 0 and 60 per cent with a median of 5 per cent [101].

Technical redescriptions of certain moral problems are necessary within the framework of ethics analysed here, because it makes it possible to discuss certain types of problem without acknowledging that the patients' interests are being directly weighed against the interests of others. Within this framework, it is difficult to discuss these problems in a more straightforward way, because that would entail a breach of the presumption that the patient and the patient's interests are of paramount importance. It is, of course, possible to advocate for a specific patient group in the abstract, and claim that they are not given sufficient priority, but a choice between individual patients that was really seen as not based solely on medical reasons is very difficult to make room for in the framework. If justice could be redescribed as a virtue or as a professional obligation in the way May suggests [102], this problem could probably be alleviated.

Conclusion

The findings presented in this chapter indicate that the health care professionals studied here posses the ethical concepts that are relevant for the assessment of many of the ethical problems that occur in health care. If they are given time and opportunity to apply these principles in ethical reasoning, they do so very proficiently, albeit in a way that combines elements from deontological ethics, consequentialism, and virtue ethics. Unfortunately, time and opportunity may be exactly what is lacking in the health care setting. This may be a significant problem if it is really the case, as one of the respondents expressed it, that '*I could think for days about many of your questions*' (DSM).

Their ethical framework inherently contains the problem areas described above (risk of paternalism, restriction of scope to the individual patient), but these problem areas only affect reasoning about certain classes of problem.

With regard to ethical perception the conclusions must be more guarded, partly because our ideas about what constitutes optimal ethical perception are more vague, partly because it seems to be an area where the findings indicate that there are more substantial problems. If bad decisions about ethical problems occur in the health care system, it could primarily be caused by deficiencies in ethical perception, rather than by deficiencies in ethical reasoning.

Notes

1 With the lowest estimate of the frequency of ethical problems (5%) the chance of encountering at least one problem in fifty patients is: $1 - (1 - 0.05)^{50} = 0.923$ or 92.3%. With the higher estimate of the frequency (20%), the chance of encountering at least one problem is for all practical purposes 100%.

2 The following conventions are used in the presentation of interview transcripts in this and the following chapters: I = interviewer; R = respondent (omitted in presentation of sections where only the respondent speaks); [...] = section omitted; {...} = word or sentence omitted to ensure anonymity.

The profession and position of respondents are identified by a three-letter code (profession, position, sex): D = doctor, N = nurse; S = consultant or chief nurse, I = junior doctor or nurse, G = general practitioner; F = female, M = male. (e.g., (DSF) is a female consultant.)

References

1 Childers, E., *The Riddle of the Sands*. Ware: Wordsworth Classics, 1993 (first published 1903).
2 Murdoch, I., *The Sovereignty of Good*. London: ARK paperbacks, 1985 (first published 1970).
3 Bok, S., *Secrets – On the Ethics of Concealment and Revelation*. New York: Vintage Books, 1989.
4 Hansen, H. P., Kvalme, Orden eller Kaos. En kulturanalyse af sygeplejen til kræftpatienter. In: Ramhøj, P. (ed.), *Overvejelser og metoder i sundhedsforskningen*. København: Akademisk Forlag, 1993: pp. 104–22.
5 Hansen, H. P., Ro, regelmæssighed og renlighed i sygeplejen. *Tidsskrift for Sygeplejeforskning* 1995; 11(1): 3–20.
6 Michaelsen, J. J., På feltarbejde i hjemmesygeplejen. In: Ramhøj, P. (ed.), *Overvejelser og metoder i sundhedsforskningen*. København: Akademisk Forlag, 1993: pp. 123–42.
7 Lee, R. M., *Doing Research on Sensitive Topics*. London: Sage Publications, 1993.
8 Kimmel, A. J., *Ethics and Values in Applied Social Research*. Newbury Park, CA: Sage Publications, 1988.
9 Mitchell, R. G., *Secrecy and Fieldwork*. Newbury Park, CA: Sage Publications, 1993.
10 Beauchamp, T. L., Faden, R. R., Wallace, R. J., Walters, L. (eds), *Ethical Issues in Social Science Research*. Baltimore: The Johns Hopkins University Press, 1982.
11 Morgan, D. L., *Focus Groups as Qualitative Research*. Sage University Paper Series on Qualitative Research Methods (vol. 16). Newbury Park, CA: Sage, 1988.
12 Stewart, D. W., Shamdasani, P. N., *Focus Groups – Theory and Practice*.

Applied Social Research Methods Series (vol. 20). Newbury Park, CA: Sage, 1990.

13 Fowler, F. J., *Survey Research Methods* (2nd edn). Applied Social Research Methods Series (vol. 1). Newbury Park, CA: Sage, 1993.

14 McCracken, G. D., *The Long Interview*. Sage University Paper Series on Qualitative Research Methods (vol. 13). Beverly Hills, CA: Sage, 1988.

15 Rest, J., *Development in Judging Moral Issues*. Minneapolis: University of Minnesota Press, 1979.

16 Rest, J., Bebeau, M., Volker, J., An overview of the Psychology of Morality. In: Rest, J. (ed.), *Moral Development: Advances in Research and Theory*. New York: Praeger, 1986: pp. 1–27.

17 Marshall, C., Rossman, G. B., *Designing Qualitative Research*. Newbury Park: Sage Publications, 1989.

18 MacIntyre, A., *A Short History of Ethics*. New York: Collier Books, 1966.

19 Ketefian, S., A case study of theory development: moral behavior in nursing. *Advances in Nursing Science* 1987; 9(2): 10–19.

20 Cassidy, V. R., Oddi, L. F., Professional autonomy and ethical decision-making among graduate and undergraduate nursing majors: a replication. *Journal of Nursing Education* 1990; 30(4): 149–51.

21 Cox, J. L., Ethical decision making by hospital nurses. Unpublished Ph.D. dissertation, Wayne State University, 1985.

22 Etiske regler for læger. In: *Lægeforeningens vejviser 1995*. København: Lægeforeningens Forlag, 1995: pp. 65–6.

23 Strauss, A., Corbin, J., Grounded theory methodology – an overview. In: Denzin, N. K., Lincoln, Y. S. (eds), *Handbook of qualitative research*. London: Sage Publications, 1994.

24 Glaser, B. G., Strauss, A. L., *The Discovery of Grounded Theory*. New York: Aldine de Gruyter, 1967.

25 Glaser, B. G., *Theoretical Sensitivity*. Mill Valley, CA: The Sociology Press, 1978.

26 Strauss, A., Corbin, J., *Basics of Qualitative Research – Grounded Theory Procedures and Techniques*. Newbury Park, CA: SagePublications, 1990.

27 Holm, S., Schmidt, L., Analyse baseret på Grounded Theory. In: Lunde, I. M., Ramhøj, P. (ed.), *Humanistisk forskning i sundhedsvidenskab*. København: Akademisk Forlag, 1995: pp. 222–35.

28 Harder, I., Grounded Theory – praksisforankret teoriudvikling. In: Ramhøj, P. (ed.), *Overvejelser og metoder i sundhedsforskningen*. København: Akademisk Forlag, 1993: pp. 59–72.

29 Giorgi, A., *Psychology as a Human Science*. New York: Harper and Row, 1970.

30 Giorgi, A., Sketch of a psychological phenomenological method. In: Giorgi, (ed.), *Phenomenological and psychological research*. Pittsburgh, PA: Duquesne University Press, 1985: pp. 8–22.

31 Crisham, P., Measuring moral judgment in nursing dilemmas. *Nursing Research* 1982; 30(2): 104–10.

32 Keller, M. C., Nurses responses to moral dilemmas. Unpublished Ed.D. thesis, University of South Carolina, 1985.

33 Davis, A. J., Ethical dilemmas: a survey. *The Canadian Nurse* 1988; 84(9): 56–8.

34 Beauchamp, T. L., Childress, J. F., *Principles of Biomedical Ethics* (4th edn). New York: Oxford University Press, 1994.

35 Gillon, R., *Philosophical Medical Ethics*. Chichester: John Wiley and Sons, 1986.

36 Gillon, R. (ed.), *Principles of Health Care Ethics*. Chichester: John Wiley and Sons, 1994.

37 Holm, S., American bioethics at the crossroads – a critical appraisal. *European Philosophy of Medicine and Health Care* 1994; 2(2): 6–23.

38 Holm, S., Not just autonomy – the principles of American biomedical ethics. *Journal of Medical Ethics* 1995; 21: 332–8.

39 Seedhouse, D., *Ethics: The Heart of Health Care*. Chichester: John Wiley and Sons, 1988.

40 Seedhouse, D., *Health – The Foundations for Achievement*. Chichester: John Wiley and Sons, 1986

41 Ross, W. D., *The Right and the Good*. Oxford: Oxford University Press, 1930.

42 Broad, C. D., *Five Types of Ethical Theory*. London: Routledge and Kegan Paul, 1930.

43 Hursthouse, R., *Beginning Lives*. Oxford: Basil Blackwell, 1987.

44 MacIntyre, A., *After Virtue* (2nd edn). Notre Dame, IL: Notre Dame University Press, 1984.

45 Aquinas, St T., *Summa Theologiæ* (vols. 1–60). London: Blackfriars, 1963.

46 Finnis, J., *Moral Absolutes – Tradition, Revision, and Truth*. Washington, DC: The Catholic University of America Press, 1991.

47 MacIntyre, A., *Whose Justice? Which Rationality?* London: Gerald Duckworth and Co., 1988.

48 Ruess, D. A., A comparison of ethical reasoning by health care professionals and parents of infants. Unpublished D.N.Sc. dissertation, The Catholic University of America, 1987.

49 Grisez, G., Boyle, J. M., *Life and Death with Liberty and Justice*. Notre Dame: Notre Dame University Press, 1979.

50 Brown, G., Yule, G., *Discourse Analysis*. Cambridge: Cambridge University Press, 1983.

51 Lunde, I. M., Om udvælgelsesstrategier i kvalitativ forskning. In: Ramhøj, P. (ed.), *Overvejelser og metoder i sundhedsforskningen*. København: Akademisk Forlag, 1993: pp. 73–81.

52 McCracken, G. D., *The Long Interview*. Sage University Paper Series on Qualitative Research Methods (vol. 13). Beverly Hills, CA: Sage Publications, 1988.

53 Malterud, K., *Allmenpraktikerens møte med kvinnlige pasienter*. Bergen: Tano, 1990.

54 Kuzel, A. J., Sampling in qualitative inquiry. In: Crabtree, B. F., Miller, W. L. (eds), *Doing Qualitative Research*. Newbury Park, CA: Sage Publications, 1992: pp. 31–44.

55 Sommerlund, B., *Textbase Alpha*. Risskov: Psykologisk Institut, 1989.

56 Pfaffenberger, B., *Microcomputer Applications in Qualitative Research.* Sage University Paper Series on Qualitative Research Methods (vol. 14). Newbury Park, CA: Sage Publications, 1988.

57 Glaser, B. G., *Basics of Grounded Theory Analysis.* Mill Valley, CA: The Sociology Press, 1992.

58 Robrecht, L. C., Grounded theory: evolving methods. *Qualitative Health Research* 1995; 5: 169–77.

59 Stern, P. N., Eroding grounded theory. In: Morse, J. M. (ed.), *Critical Issues in Qualitative Research Methods.* Thousand Oaks, CA: Sage Publications, 1994: pp. 212–23.

60 Miles, M. B., Huberman, A. M., *Qualitative Data Analysis: An Expanded Sourcebook* (2nd edn). Thousand Oaks, CA: Sage, 1994.

61 Fisher, A., *The Logic of Real Arguments.* Cambridge: Cambridge University Press, 1988.

62 Fogelin, R. J., Sinnott-Armstrong, W., *Understanding Arguments – An Introduction to Informal Logic* (4th edn). New York: Harcourt Brace Jovanovich Publishers, 1991.

63 Walton, D. N., *Informal Logic – A Handbook for Critical Argumentation.* Cambridge: Cambridge University Press, 1989.

64 Walton, D. N., *Plausible Argument in Everyday Conversation.* Albany: State University of New York Press, 1992.

65 Kuhn, D., *The Skills of Argument.* Cambridge: Cambridge University Press, 1991.

66 Åqvist, L., Deontic logic. In: Gabbay, D., Guenthner, F. (eds), *Handbook of Philosophical Logic* (vol II). Dordrecht: D. Reidel Publishing Company, 1984: pp. 605–714.

67 Gowans, C. W. (ed.), *Moral Dilemmas.* Oxford: Oxford University Press, 1987.

68 Geach, P. (ed.), *Logic and Ethics.* Dordrecht: Kluwer Academic Publishers, 1991.

69 Austen, J., *Pride and Prejudice.* Ware: Wordsworth Classics, 1992 (first published 1813).

70 Blum, L., Moral perception and particularity. *Ethics* 1991; 101(4): 701–25.

71 Jonas, H., *The Imperative of Responsibility – In Search of an Ethics for the Technological Age.* Chicago: University of Chicago Press, 1984.

72 Kollemorten, I., Strandberg, C., Thomsen, B. M., Wiberg, O., Windfeld-Schmidt, T., Binder, V., Ethical aspects of clinical decision-making. *Journal of Medical Ethics* 1981; 7: 67–9.

73 Holm, S., Röck, N. D., Sørensen, L., Ibsen, K. E. M., Etiske problemer i skadestuearbejdet. *Ugeskrift for Læger* 1993; 155(39): 3112–14.

74 Davis, A. J., Ethical dilemmas in nursing: a survey. *Western Journal of Nursing Research* 1981; 3(4): 397–407.

75 Hébert, P., Meslin, E. M., Dunn, E. V., Byrne, N., Reid, S. R., Evaluating ethical sensitivity in medical students: using vignettes as an instrument. *Journal of Medical Ethics* 1990; 16: 141–5.

76 Stevens, N. G., McCormick, T. R., What are students thinking when we present ethics cases? an example focusing on confidentiality and substance

abuse. *Journal of Medical Ethics* 1994; 20: 112–7.

77 Parfit, D., *Reasons and Persons*. Oxford: Oxford University Press, 1984.

78 Ross, W. D., *Foundations of Ethics*. Oxford: Oxford University Press, 1939.

79 Becker, H. S., Geer, B., Hughes, E. C., Strauss, A. L., *Boys in White – Student Culture in Medical School*. Chicago: University of Chicago Press, 1961.

80 Aristotle, Ethics. London: Penguin Classics, 1976.

81 Buber, M., *I and Thou* (2nd edn). Edinburgh: T and T Clark, 1987 (original in German 1923).

82 Brody, H., *The Healer's Power*. New Haven, CT: Yale University Press, 1992.

83 Ajzen, I., Attitude structure and behavior. In: Breckler, S. J., Greenwald, A. G. (eds), *Attitude Structure and Function*. Hillsdale, NJ: Lawrence Erlbaum, 1989: pp. 241–74.

84 Gorsuch, R. L., Ortberg, J., Moral obligation and attitudes: their relation to behavioral intentions. *Journal of Personality and Social Psychology* 1983; 44: 1025–8.

85 Randall, D. M., Gibson, A. M., Ethical decision making in the medical profession: an application of the theory of planned behavior. *Journal of Business Ethics* 1991; 10: 111–22.

86 Omery, A. K., The moral reasoning of nurses who work in the adult intensive care setting. Unpublished D.N.Sc. dissertation, Boston University, 1985.

87 Lützén, K., *Moral Sensitivity; A Study of Subjective Aspects of the Process of Moral Decision Making in Psychiatric Nursing*. Stockholm: Karolinska Institutet, 1993.

88 Udén, G., Norberg, A., Lindseth, A., Marhaug, V., Ethical reasoning in nurses' and physicians' stories about care episodes. *Journal of Advanced Nursing* 1992; 17: 1028–34.

89 Moe, C., *Plejehjemsbeboeres ønsker vedrørende det lægelige behandlingssigte ved livstruende sygdom – En medicinsk-humanistisk undersøgelse*. København: Lægeforeningens Forlag, 1995.

90 Gundelach, P., Riis, O., *Danskernes Værdier*. København: Forlaget Sociologi, 1992.

91 Williams, B., A critique of utilitarianism. In: Smart J. J. C., Williams, B., *Utilitarianism – For and Against*. Cambridge: Cambridge University Press, 1973: pp. 77–150.

92 Dancy, J., *Moral Reasons*. Oxford: Blackwell Publishers, 1993.

93 Wulff, H. R., Pedersen, S. A., Rosenberg, R., *Philosophy of Medicine – An Introduction*. Oxford: Blackwell Publishers, 1986.

94 Nussbaum, M. C., *Love's Knowledge – Essays on Philosophy and Literature*. New York: Oxford University Press, 1990.

95 Graber, G. C., Thomasma, D. C., *Theory and Practice in Medical Ethics*. New York: Continuum Publishing, 1989.

96 Thomasma, D. C., Pellegrino, E. D., Philosophy of medicine as the source for medical ethics. *Metamedicine* 1981; 2: 5–11.

97 Gorovitz, S., *Doctors' Dilemmas: Moral Conflict and Medical Care*. New York: Macmillan Publishers, 1982.

98 Burke, G. B., Ethics and medical decision-making. *Primary Care* 1980; 7(4): 615–24.

99 Wulff, H. R., The inherent paternalism in clinical practice. *The Journal of Medicine and Philosophy* 1995; 20: 299–311.

100 Weston, A., Toward a social critique of bioethics. *Journal of Social Philosophy* 1991; 22(2): 109–18.

101 Van McCrary, S., Swanson, J. W., Youngner, S. J., Perkins, H. S., Winslade, W. J., Physicians' quantitative assessment of medical futility. *The Journal of Clinical Ethics* 1994; 5(2): 100–5.

102 May, W. F., The virtues in a professional setting. In: Fulford, K. W. M., Gillett, G., Soskice, J. M. (eds), *Medicine and Moral Reasoning*. Cambridge: Cambridge University Press, 1994: pp. 75–90.

5

Ethical decision-making and the organisation of health care delivery

An organization is a collection of choices looking for problems, issues and feelings looking for decision situations in which they might be aired, solutions looking for issues to which they might be the answers, and decision-makers looking for work. [James G. March, cited from 1, p. 117]

All who work in public administration are constantly confronted with ethical decisions. These decisions are just as important as those that deal with other issues in the administration, for instance the effectivenes of the enterprise, its rationality, or its legality. They are maybe even more important since, in a fundamental way, they affect the relationship between human beings both within and outside of the bureaucracies. The legitimacy of a regime can be directly dependent upon its ethical standard. In other words, the citizens do not in the long run accept an unethical system. (my translation from the original Swedish) [2, p. 7]

Introduction

The ethical decision-making of individual health care professionals does not occur in a vacuum. It is influenced by attitudes in society at large, by the general social environment in which the professional lives, and by the organisational features of the health care institution in which the professional works.

Danish health care professionals working in hospitals are all salaried public employees, and have to combine a professional role with a bureaucratic role. The limits of the health care they deliver is not only decided by their own standards and the size of the patient's bank account; the organisation imposes limits, which the health care professional is supposed to uphold as a loyal employee. Even though general practitioners are, in principle, not employees but free-standing contractors, the reality is that their contract with the health services is so detailed and specific that they also have to take on part of the bureaucratic role.

These organisational features of health care delivery in Denmark mean that many of the classic analyses of the medical profession, such as Freidson's *Profession of Medicine* [3], and many of the classic hospital studies are inapplicable because they take their point of departure in a health care system where most professionals are working in individual fee-for-service practice. Likewise, many studies of organisational features of hospitals carried out in the 1970s are now obsolete, because of the rapid changes in hospital structure [4].

In the previous chapter I developed an account of the moral reasoning of health care personnel centred around a core notion of 'protective responsibility'. In this chapter I want to explore how the organisation of the health care system influences the ethical decision-making process, to examine what happens when ethical disagreement occurs, and to look at how the professional and the bureaucratic roles become integrated. I will mainly focus on the areas where the study identifies problems, since these are the areas where organisational change could be warranted.

The organisation of hospitals – structure, process, culture

In organisational theory it is common to employ a distinction between structure, process, and culture, and to describe the influence of these three separate factors on decision-making (see Figure 5.1 [5]. In the following short overview I will try to follow that approach, although my aim is not a full account of the organisation of hospitals.

Seen from the point of view of health care professionals,

Figure 5.1 Influences of organisation

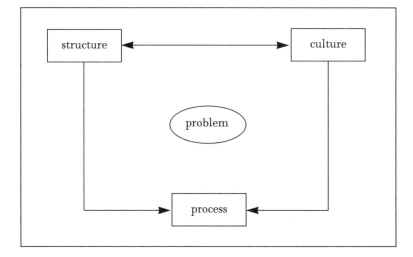

the basic structural unit of the hospital is the department, and, along with their professional group, it is the main point of identification for hospital personnel. When asked where they come from most will answer something like: 'I am senior registrar in the department of cardiology.' Other departments in the same hospital, and the hospital administration, are usually seen as outsiders.

The internal structure of the department varies between different hospital departments, but doctors and nurses are usually organised in two parallel hierarchies with separate line-management structures that are only directly related at the overall departmental management level (see Figure 5.2). This formal structure is similar to that in the other Nordic countries [6], and it agrees with the three different leadership models developed by Eriksen and Larsen [7], who, in their analysis of a large Norwegian hospital, identified a hierarchical model, a professional model, and a team model. In the hierarchical model the chief consultant had assumed power, in the professional model physicians and nurses each took care of their own problems, and only in the team model was there real cooperation between the two groups at the administrative level. This

Figure 5.2 The management structure of a 'typical' Danish hospital department

	hospital director
	chief nurse
	chief physician
Nurses	*Doctors*
chief nurse	chief consultant
deputy chief nurse	consultants
	senior registrars
nurses	house staff
assistant nurses	

linear picture of the organisation is an abstraction, and it could lead one to believe that hospital departments are paradigm models of a Weberian bureaucracy with a strict hierarchical structure, and explicit rules for what decisions can be made at a given level in the hierarchy. The reality is, however, much more complicated.

First, there are extensive interchanges of information, requests, and orders between nurses and physicians at all levels. Physicians can order a nurse to initiate or end treatments, but the nurse has a separate personal legal responsibility as a certified health professional and must ascertain that a given prescription is reasonable and appropriate. In practice, this gives nurses a certain latitude with regard to the way in which prescriptions are carried out, although it may also create legal problems when nurses change treatments without prior consultation with a physician [8, 9]. In the sociological literature three possible relationships are outlined between a dominant profession (in this case doctors) and an allied occupation (in this case nurses); subordination, limitation, and exclusion. The relationship between doctors and nurses (as professional groups) is traditionally conceptualised as one of subordination, where all responsibility is delegated from doctors, and the possibility for autonomous decision-making is limited [10]. This model does not, however, seem to fit the present situation, in which the increasing professionalisation of nursing and the establishment of an independent knowledge base, have led to a more complex relationship. Second the hierarchical structure is only fully functioning between 8 a.m. and 4 p.m. During evening and night shifts subordinate staff have much greater latitude to make and implement decisions. Third, nodal decision-making points may appear at any time, and at any level in the hierarchy. There are no strict mechanisms ensuring either the identification of decisions that should be taken, or that specific types of decisions will always be taken at an appropriate level in the hierarchy. These three factors taken together indicate that the structure is not a Weberian rational bureaucracy, despite initial appearances to the contrary.

Because the real structure is so complex decision-making is also complicated. The classical models for rational administrative behaviour cannot be followed [11], and it would probably be correct to say that hospital departments to a large extent function by the 'garbage can model of organisational choice' [12]. According to this model, problems, solutions, participants, and choices meet at random during the workings of the organisation. Decisions are made when they all coincide. Although the individual decision may be a rational decision and may resolve the problem, the process is not in itself rational. If, for instance, we imagine a situation in which the chief nurse of the department believes that discipline has become slack, and that he or she will have to do something, he or she may decide severely to reprimand the next person who is late for work. In this sense a problem has been identified, a choice has already been made, a solution has been chosen, and the pre-made decision just awaits the confluence of the appropriate situation and the appropriate participants.

In hospital departments steps are taken to try to ensure that problems and participants meet, so that choices can be made. This is the function of ward rounds and of the various formal or informal conferences within and between the two professional groups. These strategies are not always successful, and patients and decisions may fall through cracks in the system.

The complex decision-making procedures suggest that the distinction between chief and leader can have some application within the hospital departments. It is not always the person with the formal organisational position (the chief) who is also the leader [13].

The organisational culture of hospitals is difficult to describe briefly, partly because each professional group has its own culture [14], and partly because the culture varies within subgroups of each profession (e.g., both psychiatrists and orthopaedic surgeons belong to the medical profession, but they have different professional cultures). In his seminal studies of work-related attitudes within a large multinational firm with a strong corporate culture (IBM), Hofstede found large national differences in attitudes towards power-distance, uncertainty avoidance, individualism, and masculinity, despite the active attempts to create a single international corporate culture [15]. He found that Denmark, the other Nordic countries, and the Netherlands were characterised by low power-distance, low uncertainty avoidance, high individualism, and low masculinity. This is also reflected in the culture of hospitals. Status differences are not as clearly marked as in Great Britain and the USA, and guidelines are usually not seen as rigid rules. The culture is more conducive to leadership by negotiation than to leadership by dictate.

In an empirical study of the culture among hospital administrators, doctors, and nurses, Eriksen and Ulrichsen found marked differences on a number of dimensions, and some of these are important for ethical reasoning and decision-making (see Table 5.1) [Modified from 14, p. 63]. These three different cultures are remarkably similar to those described by Kinnunen in his studies of cultures and subcultures in a Finnish polyclinic. He identified a medical culture based on science and specialisation, a nursing culture based on direct patient contact, caring, and a strong group identity, and an administrative culture based on a generalist identity [16].

Table 5.1   Organisational culture of health care personnel

Dimensions	Administrator	Doctor	Nurse
human relations	individualistic, competitive	individualistic, competitive	group-oriented
human activity	decisive, active	decisive, active	process-oriented, active
truth and reality	rational/legal	technological/ scientific	rational/ scientific, intuition
relation to the environment	dominating, generalist	dominating, specialist	seeking harmony, generalist
core mission	economy	patient/research	patient/own group
human nature	neutral, changeable	neutral, changeable	good, changeable

This short introduction to the structure, processes, and culture of hospital departments has focused on the organisation as it is experienced by employees. Seen from the point of view of the patients the picture is quite different, and other groups than doctors and nurses become salient [17]. Because the focus of this work is the ethical decision-making of doctors and nurses, I will, however, continue primarily to use the perspective of the health care professionals.

Staff structure and ethical process

Before the initiation of the present study, I held the hypothesis that the medical hierarchy and staff structure of hospitals had a major negative influence on the resolution of ethical problems, but the analysis of the data indicates that this is probably not the case. Most of the doctors interviewed think that the present medical staff structure causes a lot of problems, especially because it is difficult to achieve continuity in patient care, but they do not think that it influences ethical decision-making in any consistently negative way. Analysis of other sections of the interviews supports this contention, and I will therefore quickly move to more important problem areas.

Time and external pressure

Many respondents mention lack of time, and external pressure to perform/produce, as the main organisational problems affecting ethical decision-making. That health care personnel feel they lack the necessary time to care optimally for patients is nothing new. The problem has been mentioned in books on medical sociology for a long time [3, 18], and it is well known that excessive performance pressure is a strong negative determinant of job satisfaction among health care workers [19].

In the preceeding chapter the analysis of ethical perception indicated that time constraints may lead to impaired perception of the ethical components of problems in two ways; by raising the threshold for the recognition of the problem, and by inducing the professional to neglect the problem without further deliberation. Work pressure over longer periods of time is also likely to lead to routinisation of perception or to ethical burn-out. In this section I want to point out that time constraints and busyness are also important in the phase where problems have been perceived and a solution is sought.

Any kind of deliberation takes time, and the time required increases when one moves away from specific guidelines and rules of thumb to modes of deliberation taking account of a greater number of features of the situation. This is also true of ethical deliberation, but because this involves the introduction of yet another facet of considerations, in addition to the technical considerations that are usually prominent, it may be especially hard hit during busy work periods:

> It takes some, you are under more pressure when you are on call, because, or at least in the department where I work we have a very large flow of patients, a typical Danish department of medicine, where people are arriving all the time, there you suddenly have an

enormous number of patients, whom you have to evaluate and consider who should be treated first, what is most important. There you often have a moral or an ethical problem, even if it is the same, you feel more pressure when you are on call and during the night. (DIM)

I think that the working conditions of doctors are not suitable. There is no time allocated to this issue, it does not receive a high priority, and due to the time constraints of daily work there is no opportunity to go deeper with the issues. You handle the problems in the order in which they appear. But the more general discussions about how you should act next time or what attitude you should have to the issue ... We have had these discussion about the law, I have to say that there have been much discussion about the law since it was changed in 1989. But otherwise there is no opportunity to – I don't know whether there is even time to discuss such issues? (DIF)

I think that you can quickly loose the ethical angle on things in your daily life, but you don't have to be forced to an extreme before you act differently, the same person acts totally different. It can be economic incentives or the work-load. (DGM)

A lot of it is a question of time, I think. Out of the corner of your eye you can just manage to see, oh, oh there could be something there, you could go into the ethics of it, you ought to do it, but simply because of lack of time you just have to act. It may be something as simple as washing a patient in bed, do you put the screens up, how do you give the bedpan, are there relatives in the room, and things like that. You know that what you are doing right now is wrong. But you may have 10,000 things on your mind, and then I think that the ethical, the moral, is the first to be neglected. (NIF)

This is not a problem that can be solved just by increasing the ethical awareness of health care professionals. In situations where time constraints are severe, it is almost inevitable that people will revert from substantial deliberation to well-tested rules of thumb or technical recipes which give an immediate answer. There are good arguments for such a strategy, and it is probably possible to show that it is the rational thing to do. If time constraints cannot be removed, the task must therefore be to make sure that ethical considerations are incorporated at an earlier stage, when rules of thumb, technical recipes, and departmental guidelines are formulated, disseminated, and absorbed. In other words, in the initial stages of socialisation of the professional, when the first rules of thumb are presented. The persistence of those early rules can perhaps best be illustrated by a quote from a general practitioner in her mid-40s with seventeen years experience as a doctor, who was contemplating not performing a barium enema X-ray on a patient who was old and frail:

> *Another situation I can remember was with a very old lady, who was just lying in her bed, and where I without doubt felt a, where I felt a tumor of the colon in this very thin old lady. I, and everyone else, agreed that it was best for her to close her eyes, and her sole remaining relative, a sister, also agreed with us that she should be spared any more suffering. But even then, I am in a situation where I say to myself, is it defensible if I do not get absolutely certain knowledge, because a long time ago, when I worked in the department of radiology, I was taught that this is a diagnosis you always have to make based on certain knowledge. (DGF)*

The external pressure, and the necessity to make decisions about priorities between patients is also felt by general practitioners. They, however, also have a distinct type of problem, because they have to negotiate on behalf of their patients with the social services, and with hospital departments:

> *I think that the work-load is too large, and that there are some things I do not see every time. (DGM)*

> *Now you ask, I have had this problem a couple of times with elderly people, where I would say, this old lady, she cannot cope at home, she ought not to be alone in her home. Sometimes she is in the hospital for social reasons, and then came to the local nursing home, where they wanted her to be in her own home with maximal home care. I did not think that she could manage, and the physiotherapists and occupational therapists thought the same, so we were very much in agreement, but we did not decide. It was the statements from the nurses in the nursing home that decided that she was allowed to move back home and fracture her hip. Now she is in the nursing home with a bad hip. I found it very frustrating to be proven right. It is not just a single incident, there are some situations where nobody listens to you. It has happened several times, and I have discussed it with the occupational therapists and physiotherapists several times, and we have said that there are times when you do not listen to us. But there are obviously also economic considerations at play. (DGF)*

The problems identified here are similar to those found by Launsø and Jensen in a large study of the working conditions and satisfaction of general practitioners [20].

Conferring with others

A substantial amount of working time in medicine and nursing is spent talking to other health professionals. How important this is varies from specialty to specialty, but especially in internal medicine, paediatrics and psychiatry the patient's case is often constructed through a discourse between professionals. This is an area of medical work which has not received much attention in medical sociology, or in medical decision-making theory [21]. The literature about how doctors or nurses talk to or with patients is very large, but studies about how they talk to each other are not very numerous. There are actually so few of these studies that a recent British author feels justified in stating:

> The naive observer, who had access only to mainstream sociological research, could all too readily assume that medical work was a predominantly solitary affair that occurred within the consulting rooms of family practitioners and their hospital counterparts. [21, p .34]

In the present project I was interested in how the possibilities of discussing the patient and the problems encountered in care and treatment influenced ethical decision-making subject that was discussed with all respondents.

The levels of conferences[1]

If an individual health care professionals encounter problems that they do not feel comfortable in deciding themselves, there are at least five options open to them within the organisational scheme:

1. ignore the problem or decide to solve it without conferring;
2. confer with a person from outside the system;
3. confer with a colleague at the same hierarchical level;
4. confer with a superior;
5. take the problem to a departmental conference.

Many departments have guidelines specifying that clinical problems of certain kinds must be referred to a specific hierarchical level before a decision can be made. For those kinds of problems junior staff have a duty to confer with superiors, but informal and formal conferring may concern all kinds of problem. Few departments have specific guidelines about referral of ethical problems, except in psychiatry where ethics and law are so intricately mixed that it is difficult to separate the ethical and the legal aspects of problems about information and procedures for involuntary admission. In daily work there are also many ethical problems that fall outside the formal guidelines, and where the person is free to choose between the five options outlined above. All five options are used to some extent, but choice is influenced by many different factors including the nature of the problem, time constraints, and departmental culture.

There is an obvious difference in the degree of formality, and the requirement for adherence to the advice/order given when one moves from the second to the fifth option. Advice from a colleague can be disregarded, whereas advice from superiors or decisions made at a departmental conference will usually have to be followed. In the following section I shall try to discuss the function of the different levels of conferencing and their importance for ethical decision-making in hospital departments. General practitioners also confer with others, when they face difficult problems, but because they are finally responsible for the treatment of their own patients, all their conferences follow the second and third options, and result in advice that they may reject.

Many respondents discuss ethical problems with people from outside the health care sector, or with colleagues who are not employed at the same department. These discussions fall in two different categories. The first is the discussion of exciting, dramatic, or interesting cases, and may occur whenever health care professionals meet. Such discussions rarely amount to more than a recounting of the interesting case, and a short exchange of opinions. Their purpose is either just to tell an interesting story, or in some cases to vent steam. The second category is discussions with family or close friends. These are usually much more intense, and centre around problems that have affected the nurse or doctor in some personal way. The purpose is usually to gain emotional support and/or real advice:

R: *We do discuss these issues, for instance when we meet with colleagues for coffee.*

I: *What kind of problems are then raised, the ordinary, the important, or the dramatic?*

R: *Well, most often the dramatic, recent problems that we talk about but which then often turn into something more general – what should be done about this, or should we generally act in this way or in that.* (DSM)

Well, then I would probably use my network of people, whom I use as advisers. My network primarily consists of my family, brothers and wives and such people, also when it concerns professional problems, if it is an ethical problem, but also the colleagues I feel most at ease with, I use them as advisers. (DIM)

What could be called 'lateral' consultations with colleagues at the same hierarchical level are also very common. They usually involve a mixture of three different questions: 'what would you do?', 'what do we usually do in cases such as this?', and 'what would you advise me to do?'. Among nurses, this kind of conference can also be initiated to gain emotional support, to create coherence in the group of nurses, or to develop a strategy before presenting the problem to a doctor:

I would talk with my colleagues. I think that such a discussion could be a good idea, and could solve the problem. It might also be the case that I was wrong. I think that collaboration is simply the most important thing. (NSF)

A study of residents in American paediatric training programmes have shown that residents most often turn to superiors (attendings) for assistance and support in resolving ethical dilemmas, but that they rate the advice and support they get from other residents and from their own spouses higher than that they get from attendings [22]. The authors hypothesise that this is caused by the attendings being 'distant', but it may as well be that attendings cannot see the problems from the point of view of the residents.

Asking a superior has both advantages and disadvantages. The advantage is that the responsibility for making a decision is put on somebody else, and that the decision can be made by somebody with more experience and knowledge; the disadvantage is that one may not agree with the decision (but see 'The tactics of conferences' below). In some instances the nurses caring for a specific patient will also initiate or be involved in conferences at this level.

Finally, full-scale departmental conferences have the advantage that a given problem can be discussed in a larger forum, and even if no real discussion takes place the conference will at least result in an authoritative decision. Older doctors also see departmental conferences as a forum for educating their younger colleagues and inculcating the correct medical culture. Some see this as a more important function of the conferences than discussion of ethical problems, which is perceived as futile. This last attitude is connected to a kind of ethical subjectivism:

> *The reason why it is not brought up at conferences is that it is the more technical, there has to be a decision, and ethics and morality are more concerned with attitudes, it is something that influences the decisions we make. But it is not something where you can decide that it should be this way or that way, whether a convention should be this way or that way, it is something intangible, something you feel, that's the way it is, you do it this way or you don't.* (DIM)

Some problems are seen as unsuitable for a formal departmental conference. These include problems that touch upon religious issues, problems involving members of staff personally (that is, not solely in their professional role), and problems that are feared to create an emotional response. These problems are perceived as more suitable for a smaller forum.

A possible disadvantage in raising ethical problems at departmental conferences is that such a discussion almost necessarily will involve people who have no personal knowledge of the patient or the problem:

Because the problem at a conference is that we are sitting there without the patient. Often there will be some present who haven't seen the patient for the last four days, and they discuss with two who have seen the patient, and if there is disagreement and differences of opinion we easily slide into something distorted, because some are sitting with a wrong set of premises. (DSM)

The patient may disappear as a person, and just become a medical problem. This worry is compatible with the data presented by Anspach, who studied case presentations in formal conference settings, and found that they are characterised by a constant rhetorical form involving both a certain order of presentation, and a certain style [23]. In order of presentation the medical history comes first, followed by the present medical problems, and then, as the last item, social aspects may be mentioned. Anspach interprets this order in the following way:

> Because social aspects of the case are always presented (if at all) only after medical problems have been discussed, the semantic structure of the base presentation attests to the relatively low priority accorded to social issues in the reward structure of residency programs. [23, p. 361]

With regard to style Anspach identifies four major characteristics: depersonalisation of the patient, omission of the agent, treating medical technology as the agent, and using 'account markers' to emphasise the subjectivity of the patient's account. The present study contains no direct observation of conferences, only reports from participants, but these give some indication of whether ethical issues are treated with the same neglect as the social issues in Anspach's material.

The analysis of the interviews shows clearly that ethical problems are seen as a separate category, which is only pertinent for discussions of some patients in specific situations. Ethical problems are not discussed for all patients, but the chance of a problem being discussed grows with the severity of the problem. A recent Danish survey showed that in discussions about termination of treatment, about 33 per cent of a sample of internists believed that ethical considerations would get the largest place in the conference discussion, 12 per cent believed that technical considerations would be dominant, and 55 per cent believed that the two aspects would get equal consideration. The same study showed that 89 per cent would raise the discussion at a conference, if they 'discovered' the problem during ward rounds [24].

The conclusion about whether ethical issues get a sufficient hearing will therefore depend on what view one takes on the frequency and severity of such issues. Should they be explicitly mentioned in each case presentation, or only when they are of sufficient severity? I tend to believe, that although the person presenting the case, and the other participants in the conference, should actively look for its ethical components, this does not necessarily lead to the conclusion that ethical issues should be mentioned in each presentation. Otherwise, we might just institute a new medical ritual where most presentations end with the invocation 'and there are no major ethical problems in this case'.

It is, however, also important not to forget that the possibility of influencing, what kinds of problem are discussed as ethical problem, is a form of power, namely to control a separate kind of discourse. And this power can be used to produce a decision-making situation which is conducive to certain kinds of decisions.

The tactics of conferences

There are also indications in the data that, although most respondents are satisfied with their *possibilities* of conferring with others, the actual *function* of the conference system does not resolve all ethical problems, and it may even create some new.

In most cases the person identifying a problem also has an opinion about its solution. If that person believes that the solution is correct ethically and/or technically, he or she will have an interest in promoting it during the conference. And if some other solution is chosen, he or she may feel compelled to show discontent in some way, especially if the solution infringes on her or his sense of responsibility towards the patient (see the section 'Exit, voice, obstruction, and loyalty' below).

Promoting a specific solution can be done openly by presenting arguments at the conference, but it can also be done covertly. There are two tactics that can be employed: choosing a suitable conference forum, and preparing and presenting the case in an appropriate form. In many cases there is a choice between different conference forums. If, for instance, there is a need to consult with superiors, most departments usually have a number of consultants, and junior staff and nurses will quickly learn which one to approach to get the desired answer, and how to present the case:

> My ethical problems are very much related to the treatment problems we have, where are we, and what can and should we do. I know these questions well enough to know with whom I want to discuss them, and you will quickly find people where you feel that you can discuss the issues in a reasonable way, get a discussion, a dialogue going, and get the qualified questioning which makes you think of some aspects of the case you might not have seen before. And then there are other people where you wouldn't raise the issue, because it would be totally trivialized, or you would get a rash decision that you don't feel you can walk away with. (DIM)

> One of the things which happens is that we in the nursing staff very quickly discover which doctors are suitable in specific situations. There may be a doctor who is incredibly good in one situation and whom we can't use at all in another situation. And we know in advance whom we should approach. (NSM)

> I think that everything ought to be discussed, but I also think that you can be in places where the attitudes are such that you don't raise all issues in order not to have some decision imposed which you are not interested in seeing imposed. Yes, I think that it can be that way. (DIF)

> In the places where I have been it has depended on the way you present the problem. This means that you present it in a way, well, you give the information, which points in the direction you want the decision to go. I think that this is often the case, and it is not a problem. (DIF)

A second type of problem is caused by the fact that there is no rational mechanism for selecting which problems or cases are discussed at the highest conference level, and thereby no mechanism ensuring that decisions about departmental policy are influenced by the 'right' sort of information. It is clear that the magnitude of a given problem (or perhaps more accurately the salience of the problem) will have an impact on whether or not it is brought up at a conference, but there is also a great element of random selection depending on extraneous factors like time constraints, 'collision' with other problems, etc.:

> *I don't think it is a specific type of problem, I think that you but I am really not in a position to say but I think that you choose relatively randomly, you choose some where you really spend time, spend time on having them thoroughly discussed and on finding a solution which is as good as possible. And that time, it is expensive with all these people around a conference table, so you have to defend it by saying that it hopefully benefits other decisions, where you don't spend as much time.* (DSM)

Finally, departmental culture seems to determine whether or not it is really possible to discuss ethical problems as such, or whether they are discussed as technical problems. Some respondents felt that ethics was given great weight in the conferences at their department, whereas others described the exact opposite situation. An initially plausible explanation for this difference could be cultural differences between specialties, but there is no support for this explanation in the present data. There is some evidence that a single strong person placed at the top of the hierarchy may have a very large influence on whether ethics is discussed or not:

> *It is evident that some places the leadership is so strong, that is, there is so strong a hierarchy in the department that it suppresses the perception of the ethical problems which other doctors or other members of the staff have, they simply do not dare to put it forward – and that is unfortunate. But in that case I don't think it is the staff structure, but more that there are individual persons who are so domineering or so authoritarian in their behaviour, that they scare people away.* (DSM)

Concluding evaluation of the possibilities for ethical discussion

If all aspects of the possibilities to discuss ethical problems with colleagues and get ethical advice are put in the balance,

the conclusion must be, first, that the structure contains sufficient discussion possibilities, second, that the local departmental culture decides whether these possibilities are utilised, and
third, that a negative attitude from consultants and chiefs of
departments may prevent proper discussions.

The last point connects with recent discussions in the management literature about the dangers of charismatic leadership
[25]. Charismatic leadership can often lead to great success
because it inspires subordinates to become followers, and
thereby to become personally interested in the success of the
organisation. But there is also a possible darker side. An 'ideal-
type' of the unethical charismatic leader has been described
with the following characteristics:

1. uses power only for personal gain or impact;
2. promotes own personal vision;
3. censures critical or opposing views;
4. demands own decisions be accepted without question;
5. one-way communication;
6. insensitive to followers' needs;
7. relies on convenient external moral standards to satisfy
    self-interest.
[modified from 25, p. 45]

Leaders of this kind do occur in health care, and even the best
organisational structure cannot protect against the unethical
effects of such leadership, if there are no external control
mechanisms. Any kind of charismatic leader tends to reproduce
her- or himself in the followers, and this is unfortunately also
true of the leader with ethically problematic attributes:

> *I can give you an example. We have for many years had a depart-
> ment of {…} here, and at times it has had consultants that were very
> untypical and very peculiar {…}. There have been people who have
> had great opinions about themselves, and have talked and written the
> case records in a different way than the norm has been in the hospi-
> tal system, and they have been very arrogant toward the patients and,
> from our point of view, acted in a totally unacceptable way. I have
> clearly felt that people who have been some time in that department
> begin to get the same attitude towards the patients, which is a case*

of like father like son. I think that a lot of what is done there is clearly lacking in ethics, and I think that the example of older colleagues is not unimportant. (DIM)

It is natural that leaders want to influence and change the organisation to fit their ideals. It is also natural to want to develop employees so that they fit into the leader's picture of the organisation, but it is important that the means used to accomplish these ends are themselves ethically acceptable. In general, the leader can have three problems with people in the organisation [13]. They may not want to follow, not be able to follow, not understand what is demanded. Any one person in the organisation may have any number of these characteristics. The optimal follower has none, the determined opponent has only the first, and the 'lost case' has all three. The leader's task is to remove all three obstacles hindering performance. This task can be accomplished in many ways, but only some of these are ethically acceptable (at least as first instance measures). It is, for example, generally not acceptable to fire all dissenters without trying to engage them in constructive dialogue first. It is not in itself unethical to use power, but it must be used to serve the purposes of the organisation, and not the leaders themselves [25].

The three characteristics of the problems mentioned above can also occur within the field of ethical conduct. Employees may not want to follow specific ethical guidelines, they may not be able to reason about ethics, or they may simply not understand what good ethical conduct is. In this case leaders can promote ethical awareness by making it an important feature on the public agenda of the organisation (e.g., by promoting real discussion), and by conducting themselves in a way that exemplifies what is expected. Leaders are judged by employees by a composite combination involving assessment of their personalities, roles, and actions; and the chances of inducing employees to emulate their leaders' actions increase if these actions are seen to be consistent with the expectations connected to the role [13]. In terms of ethical conduct in health care this implies that a leader who is not living up to the professional code of ethics cannot expect employees to do so either. In this context it is interesting to note that a classic study of the influence of hierarchical structure on health care outcomes shows that strongly hierarchical departments do worse in terms of productivity, patient outcome, and employee satisfaction [26, 27].

It is therefore rather problematic that (at least) American studies tend to show that mistreatment and misconduct is pervasive in medical school training, and that the students themselves think that they have become 'more cynical about academic life and the medical profession' [28, p. 533], because of these episodes. In a similar but slightly more humourous vein, British medical students talk about their pre-cynical and cynical years (instead of pre-clinical and clinical).

In management literature the concept of 'ethical climate' has been identified as an important determinant for ethical behaviour. Victor and Cullen identify the following five factors in the ethical climate of the firms they study [modified from 29, p. 112]:

1. caring (for other employees and for customers);
2. law and code (following external rules);
3. rules (following internal rules);
4. instrumental (looking out for company interests);
5. independence (using your own personal judgement).

They find that the ethical climate varies between firms, and that this variance can be explained by a) general societal norms for the specific kind of enterprise, b) organisational structure, and c) firm-specific factors. Within the hospital context, general societal norms and organisational structure do not vary much across departments, and it is therefore likely that department-specific factors are the main determinants of variation in ethical climate between hospital departments. These factors include the attitudes of the departmental leaders, and this consideration further reinforces the importance of ethical leadership.

Exit, voice, obstruction, and loyalty

As described above, there are many organisational processes for the resolution of ethical problems. Nevertheless, there are some ethical problems that cannot be resolved by argument, and where no compromise can be found. In those situations a decision will usually be made by the person with the highest hierarchical position. There are also (as described above) other situations where the leadership does not allow discussion, but simply imposes a decision. In a large number of these cases the decision will have to be carried out by somebody else (e.g., a nurse or a junior doctor). If the person who has to carry out the decision disagrees, it can create a separate ethical problem, and it places the subordinate in a difficult position within the organisation.

Hirschman has suggested a general framework for the options open to a person or group of persons who are dissatisfied with specific decisions within an organisation, or with the organisation as such [30]. He claims that there are three basic options, which he labels as 'Exit' (leave the organisation), 'Voice' (complain publicly), and 'Loyalty' (stay put and accept). This framework has later been extended by Lundquist, who shows that a fourth option – 'Obstruction' (obstruct or delay implementation) – is a possibility in many bureaucratic organisations [2]. The analysis of the data from the present study did not give rise to any better analytic categories than these four, and the data on responses to disagreement were therefore analysed within this framework.

The first finding to emerge was, that both nurses and some doctors can affect 'Exit' from a problematic situation without leaving the organisation. This option is open to nurses because they are organised in a separate hierarchy. Within that hierarchy they have to follow orders, but if they strongly disagree with an order received from a doctor, they can refuse to carry it out, and refer the physician in question to somebody higher up in the nursing hierarchy (this strategy is especially useful outside normal working hours, because no superiors will be present, and the decision must be postponed to the following day). A similar option is open to junior anaesthetists, who can refuse or delay the requests from surgeons:

> *I have refused to carry out an order. It was about giving a patient a drug. I start work and hear that a seriously ill patient, an AIDS patient, should have this. I hear that he should have a drug, and my first reaction is 'What is this drug, I have never given it before', 'Yes, it is not something we usually have and it was retracted by the Board of Health.' Well, I thought that I could look it up and read about the drug and the side-effects before I gave it to the patient, but there is nothing to be found in the large national catalogue of drugs, and nothing in the departmental instructions. I asked the chief nurse, she had never heard about it. I try to look in the patient records but it only says that it should be given in this dosage, and that the consultant will contact the Board of Health to get permission to use it. And I still don't know anything about what kind of drug it is or about the side-effects. Then I ask the house-officer, but she had never heard about it. Luckily enough it is time for evening rounds, and it is one of the more experienced physicians, so I can ask him. Well, he had not heard about it either. Then I had to tell him that I could not give the patient this drug, and he becomes very angry and takes the tablet and goes and gives it to the patient. He comes back and says that this will be a conference matter, that I have refused to give the medicine, and that he was going to talk to the chief nurse. But it turns out that you can refer to laws and paragraphs stating that I have a right to refuse, so everything turned out all right, but it was a case where I had to refuse. (NIF)*

> *I do think that as an anaesthetist you have a damned duty to hold back and react and not just let yourself be, I would almost say controlled – that is, just automatically say, OK, we give an anaesthetic, and if you say that she should be operated, we of course anaesthetise her. You have to stop and, well, sometimes it is just that we say we would like to wait for a couple of hours and use those hours to optimise the patients somatic condition, so that the chance of a positive result improves. It is often in situations like that where the surgeons come running saying 'It has to be here and now'; and where we then say, 'All right, but then we are going to kill the patient', but if we can wait for two hours, where we do this, and this, and this then we can change the prospects substantially. That is also demanding, because you have to mobilise your own opinions. (DIM)*

For the ordinary junior doctor 'Exit' is, however a very costly solution to an ethical disagreement, since only real 'Exit' – that is, leaving the department in question – is a possibility. Many junior doctors are in the middle of a training programme leading towards specialist recognition, and if they decide to leave the department they will also have to leave the training programme. It is therefore not surprising that very few mention this option when directly asked what they would do if they thought that a treatment decision was ethically very problematic.

Within the system there are a few areas where a form of internal 'Exit' is seen as legitimate. This is, for instance, the case for those people who have religious objections towards participating in abortions, and those who do not want to participate in operations on Jehova's Witnesses without access to blood transfusion. The number of instances where this right to conscientious objection can be exercised is, however, limited, and does not cover most of the areas where ethical problems can occur. It is also a question that is being increasingly scrutinised by health care administrators, who want to be certain that there really is a religious or other sufficiently weighty reason behind an objection [31].

Because 'Exit' is not seen as a realistic option, the choice of reaction has to be made between the three remaining options; and the data show that this choice in most cases is further narrowed so that only 'Loyalty' and 'Voice' are considered valid options. 'Obstruction' is only mentioned by a few, and then in connection with work in departments where some specific ethical problem is recurrent:

> I was working in the department I mentioned before, and I knew that the consultant would not, or could not do anything. The department was split in two, and what I did was, that I, for instance, when a patient was not treated who I believed could be treated, then I arranged a transferral to another hospital. But I felt that a direct confrontation, a direct discussion would only have made matters worse, so I simply tried to act, but I could only do it when it became my responsibility. In that case I did act a couple of times, but I did not have the courage to act in a more general way, and raise a case against the person in question. (DIM)

'Obstruction' can either be retroactive, as in the quote above, or pre-emptive, as described in the following quote:

What I do vis à vis the physicians is that I tell them that I cannot be controlled by what they tell me to tell the patient or not tell the patient. Because, if the patient asks me a question, then the patient has a right to an answer, and there is no one in this system who can order me to lie. [...] But if I know in advance that we are going to get problems, and we always try to be ahead of the situation. If I know that we are going to get a problem, and that this is the attitude which is going to be prevalent among the physicians, then I usually try to make sure that we have talked with the patient, opened the issue, before it reaches the conference, because then there is no way back. (NSM)

This strategy fits well with the description of the problematic situation of nurses found in Mechanic:

Good nursing care requires judgment and sensitivity and also demands that the nurse make a variety of decisions ... The authority system of care in the hospital, however, is designed to make it appear that the nurses' responses are reactive to physician judgments and orders. Thus while nurses frequently exercise important powers of decision, they must do so subtly, avoiding the appearance of being in command. [18, p. 361]

The distribution of the different reactions to disagreement is also similar to the distribution found in a quantitative survey of physicians working in departments of internal medicine [24].

Among the respondents who mention protest as a possible option, two distinctly different forms of protest can be identified. One could be called 'Internal Voice' and is defined by the fact that the protest is not communicated outside the department, whereas in the other 'External Voice' the protest is directed at people from outside the department (e.g., the administration, or the public). Very few mention 'External Voice' as a realistic option. These respondents are all consultants, and 'External Voice' is mentioned as a last resort, to be used when one has identified some systematic failure or injustice in the health care system.

'External Voice' is close to what is usually called 'whistleblowing' (that is, public exposure of problematic conditions in an organisation). There is general agreement in the theoretical literature that whistle-blowing is ethically defensible if the problem is of sufficient magnitude, and if all other avenues of action within the organisation have been exhausted without result [32, 33]. The fact that 'External Voice' is mentioned so rarely in the interviews indicates either that very few ethical problems of sufficient severity occurs to warrant 'External Voice', or that loyalty within the organisation is high, or that anyone resorting to 'External Voice' will get into trouble. The true explanation is probably a combination of these three, since there is no reason to believe that the Danish health care system is plagued by a large number of systemic ethical problems of a magnitude which require whistle-blowing.

'Internal Voice' is mentioned by most respondents, and involves the attempt to secure that the decision is not finalised, and to reverse the decision by presenting arguments for the opposite conclusion. This involves a certain degree of bias, because only the information favouring one's own position is mentioned. This strategy is used by both doctors and nurses, and is well described in the following quote:

> *If you have a different opinion you keep a keen eye on the patient, and every single thing you find to your advantage, everything which points in the other direction, you use to say, hey, that was not true, shouldn't we instead ... and then I must admit that you don't encounter resistance, so you can change a decision. But one should not forget that the decisions are most often right. But the one occasion where they are not, there you can change them. But you have to do something active, you have to act. It is not enough just to criticise, you have to present your own proposal for a solution. How should we act? Could we act differently?* (DSM)

One problem with this kind of internal protest is that it can be difficult to criticise a decision without at the same time criticising the person who has made the decision. This problem is most acute for junior staff, since the decision-maker will usually be in a more powerful position than they are themselves.

Loyalty to the group is an important part of the socialisation taking place during medical and nursing education, and there is some truth to the assertion that doctors are socialised to be 'as thick as thieves'. The organisation also maintains loyalty-promoting mechanisms, both in the form of formal and informal punishment for disloyalty, and in the form of departmental conferences. In particular, junior doctors and nurses are very conscious of the fact, that their future employment possibilities are affected by the way they behave:

> *And it is no use, when you are in a locum lasting 1, 2, or 3 months, it is no use shouting too loudly, because then your job isn't extended; and I think that many keep a very low profile, and I have done that as well in some places, because you have to do it, you don't want to be awkward.* (DIF)

> *And there are also departments where you as a nurse are told that if you cannot work under these conditions, then you can just find yourself another job elsewhere.* (NIF)

Departmental conferences promote loyalty with respect to specific decisions because they give everybody a chance to present their opinion and their arguments. In this way, participants in a departmental conference all become, at least psychologically, responsible for the final decision. Your opinion has been heard, and, although it was overruled, you have been part of a legitimate decision process, and the result of this process is in itself prima facie legitimate:

> *It is part of the rules at a place like this that if we make a conference decision, then it is a sort of dictatorship of the majority, those who are best able to argue, or it is the boss who has this attitude and decides that it should be this way. So when a decision has been made you have to be loyal, that can be difficult, but you know that you yourself would be angry, if you had been part of a decision that was not followed, if one of my colleagues just did the exact opposite because he had a different opinion, then he would have harmed that doctor–patient relationship. So in this context I would follow the decision.* (DIM)

It is evident in the data that the loyalty which is expressed is primarily loyalty towards colleagues. Loyalty towards the department is also mentioned, whereas loyalty towards the organisation as such plays no significant role, perhaps because it is seen as too remote and inaccessible:

> *The thing which is very difficult is to raise discussions with the relevant people. In these large systems you don't get to talk with the people who have designed the systems.* (DSF)

Medical errors and loyalty

The fact that loyalty towards colleagues is important is further reinforced by the responses to case 5, which describes a situation in which a colleague has made an error and thereby harmed a patient. The type of medical error described in this case falls within the group of either technical or judgemental errors as defined by Bosk in his study of the management of medical failure in an American surgical training programme [34]. Technical or judgemental errors do not reflect badly on the professional as a person, and if there is no evidence of repeated errors, the individual will be forgiven. Errors of this sort are believed to be of the kind that could happen to anyone. In contrast to these two types of error Bosk also describes normative and quasi-normative errors. These constitute breaches of the due diligence expected from a health care professional, and as a result they lead to severe professional criticism. This is true irrespective of whether or not the error leads to legal culpability for the health care professional in question.

The responses to this case in the present study are consistent with the type of responses which Bosk records for nonnormative errors. Errors are unfortunate, but we all make them now and then, and as long as the person learns from them everything is fine (what is sometimes disparagingly called the 'there but for the grace of God go I' attitude). It may be necessary to make the colleague aware of the error, but this is best handled on a one-to-one basis and not in public at a conference. But errors are noted, and when they reach what Freidson has termed a 'critical mass' [3], action is taken:

> *You have to be specific and say that if it is a single incident you can let it pass with an admonition. If there are repeated incidents it depends on the accumulated sum of incompetence for the person, and then there are various possibilities for action.* (DIM)

This action may range from a talking-to, to a disbarment from certain tasks, to the suggestion that the person finds other employment [3]. What action is chosen depends both on the severity of the errors, and on the hierarchical status of the person making them. Consultants are almost immune to such sanctions:

> *Let us say that it is a department of surgery and that the situation is becoming critical for the colleague in question, then I am of the opinion that the consultant will have to institute a partial restriction on operative procedures, so that the person in future only performs those procedures which experience has shown that he can perform. But the situation can be so intolerable that you have to free yourself from the employee in question, or to put it bluntly, dismissal.* (DIM)

> *I have experienced a single incident with someone who was not in clinical work, but worked in a paraclinical specialty, who was extremely drunk when he came to the conferences. I found that very unethical, since he should be there to advise us about what we should do with the patients in certain situation; and his word was, he was like the expert, and I found that very unethical.* (DIF)

> *Now, I am the boss. But if it is a colleague at the same level, I don't think I can do very much.* (DSM)

Bosk's study was mainly concerned with the response of hospital consultants (attendings) towards error, but the data in the present study show that the same attitude is shared by both junior and senior staff.

Bosk's study was performed in the 1970s and his informants do not at any point mention that patients ought to be, or were, informed of the medical mismanagement of their cases. This is, however, a recurrent theme in the present responses. Many respondents mention the 1990 Danish law on no-fault insurance as a major consideration, stating that the patient now has a direct monetary interest in the information, whether or not the error constitutes legal negligence. A few respondents view the problem raised by the case as a purely legal matter:

> *Now we have the new patient-insurance scheme, and there you have to, you have to inform the patient that damage has occured; and then the case is initiated. Well, it is our duty.* (DIF)

But the great majority talk about balancing the interests of an unfortunate colleague against the interests of the patient. In this balance, the possibility of receiving compensation now weighs heavily on the patient's side, along with the general presumption discussed earlier that patients have a right to know the truth about themselves.

This mode of reaction can be explained within the 'protective responsibility' framework developed in the previous chapter. Before the introduction of no-fault insurance, the individual patient had little to gain by being made aware of a possible medical error (the chance of proving negligence was small, as was the compensation awarded by the courts in succesful suits), and the responsibility of the professional to look after the best interests of the patient did not, therefore, come into operation at all, or was easily outweighed by loyalty towards a colleague. The only active responsibility was to protect future patients from harm, and this could be discharged by making the colleague aware of the error, and monitoring her or his future performance. With no-fault insurance the gain to the patient suddenly becomes much larger, and although the colleague is still at risk, the primary responsibility of protecting the best interest of the patient becomes active, and overrides both professional loyalty and a more general consequentialist analysis. The introduction of no-fault insurance has therefore activated a core component of ethical reasoning for the benefit of patients.

At the same time, responsibility towards the colleague can be discharged by offering emotional support. And because health care professionals are usually conscientious, there is a great need for support, because errors are usually taken very seriously by those who commit them:

> *The first thing I would do would be to talk to my colleague privately and say: I happened to see that you did so and so. I want to help you and support you, or something to that effect. I think that the patient must be told. I have made an error myself and it was so horrible. The only thing I could think about was that somebody had to be told, somebody had to help and support me. I informed the patient myself,*

and afterwards it was nice. It was not very pleasant but it went all right. It was not dangerous, but it was an error I had made. (NIF)

Perceived differences in ethical approach within and between the professional groups

In the previous chapter I presented an account of the ethical reasoning of health care professionals, according to which there were no major differences between workers in different specialties or between doctors and nurses. In this section I want to look at a slightly different question; what differences do health care professionals themselves perceive?

This question is of interest in the organisational context, because decisions are always made on the basis of what is perceived to be the case, and not on the basis of the case as it really is. In an organisational setting it may not matter so much whether there really is a difference between two groups, the mere perception of a difference may influence decision-making.

One of the questions put to all respondents was whether they felt they were typical in their ethical thinking compared to their professional group. Not surprisingly none of the respondents felt that their ethical thinking and attitudes were inferior to their colleagues. Most felt that they were fairly typical, and some working in psychiatry, gynaecology and obstetrics, and geriatrics felt that their specialty exposed them to so many ethical problems, that they were more ethically aware than their colleagues in other specialties:

R: *I think that I am typical among psychiatrists and that has something to do with the distinctive working conditions. There are also some with other opinions and other ethical codes etc. But I think that it is more a question that we as psychiatrists can be in opposition to or disagreement with colleagues from other specialties.*

I: *Can you specify what this difference could be?*

R: *I think that it is a question of the matter at hand. If we think about the daily work of an orthopaedic surgeon, and the daily life of a psychiatrist − that is the patients' problems − there is a different scale of magnitude − and I am certain the orthopaedic surgeon is an ethical person − but it can never be so extensive, so nuanced, so present in the mind, as among psychiatrists, that I cannot imagine.* (DSM)

Table 5.2   **Attributes of medical and nursing ethics**

Medical ethics	Nursing ethics
is masculine	is feminine
is paternal	is maternal
is linear	is circular/spiral
is hierarchical	is a web of interaction
is top-down	is bottom-up
is logical	is fuzzy-edged
is thinking-oriented	is feelings-oriented
favours theory	favours experience
its symbol is Logos	its symbol is Eros
is ruled more by the head than the heart	is ruled more by the heart than the head
starts with the self	starts with community
is introspective/egoistical	shares with others
establishes rules	recognises many predisposing conditions
establishes dilemmas	sees value conflicts
assumes responsibility for the dilemma	assumes responsibility for the choices to be made
begins with a supremely free conscience	begins with relationship and relationality
begins with a moral attitude	begins with moral reasoning
is based on principles	is based on possibilities
wants perfection	good enough is good enough
seeks solutions	seeks better understanding/to care
is aware of solitude	is aware of solidarity
results in anguish	results in joy
is detached	is attached
seeks power	seeks partnership
is directing	is nourishing
tells others what to do	listens to others' stories
is exclusive	is inclusive
is diagnosis-oriented	is person-oriented
is disease-specific	is holistic
pursues diagnosis → prognosis → treatment	is concerned with healing
is high-tech oriented	is high-touch oriented
relies heavily on the senses	relies heavily on intuition
cares from the outside	cares from the inside

In the literature on nursing ethics a sharp distinction is often made between nursing ethics, which has all the positive attributes one can think of, and medical ethics, which is cold and rationalistic. This point of view is, for instance, exemplified in Table 5.2, modified from a recent British course book in nursing ethics [35, p. 11]. As was argued in the previous chapter, the present data do not support such a strong dichotomy on the level of everyday ethical decision-making. The data does, however, indicate some differences in perception.

Most of the interviewees claim that there is a difference in the way in which nurses and doctors respond to ethical problems, but they see this not in terms of different reasoning, but in terms of different emotions. Both doctors and nurses say that nurses take their emotions more into account, and see this as a function of their closer relationship with the patient. This finding indicates that the differences between medical and nursing cultures are reproduced in the perceptions of ethical decision-making. It also points to the differences in knowledge which the different professional roles entail [36, 37]. Doctors and nurses live in different niches in the organisation, which can be understood as an 'ecology of knowledge', as Anspach has shown in her analysis of life-and-death decision-making in neonatal care: 'Each occupational group has a different set of daily experiences which define the contours of the information used in making prognostic judgements and in reaching life-and-death decisions' [36, p. 217].

Some doctors see the difference as a benefit, and believe that it leads to better decisions, whereas others think that it makes a rational assessment difficult. The same perceived difference in ethical approach is thus evaluated in two quite different ways. These two different perceptions find adherents among both consultants and junior doctors:

There can be somewhat different attitudes. The nurses who care for the patient each day and register how much or how little pain is present often have a, how shall I put it, are often a little bit quicker to propose a morphine infusion – that is, where we give a continuous infusion of morphine in a vein so that the patient's pain can be relieved, but often sedation occurs too. And the physicians are per-

haps a little more reluctant, and I think that it is because they don't see the patient as often. They come now and again and look at the patient, and then judge that now is the right time; but this judgement is, according to my experiences, in general made a little later than the nurses. Therefore we often have the problem that the younger physicians, and especially those who obviously do not yet have the same, how shall I put it, broadness in their decision-making, they say, let us wait a little more. For this reason I personally experience that I am called in by a nurse, who says, could you try to look at this case, should we or shouldn't we; and in almost all cases I agree with the nurses that the right time has come. That is the classic example. (DSM)

The nurses know more about the patients, at least those who are on the ward, because they are with the patients maybe 5–6 hours a day, at least the patients who are very ill. We are there 15 minutes during the ward round, perform some examinations, order some medicine and leave again. It is obvious that they get closer to the person, and without the input you can get from the nurses, who have a different opportunity to speak with the patient, it becomes difficult for us to evaluate, well, what is the content of the life of this patient, what is the patient's quality of life. So I think that they, in this way, have a better basis for evaluating the real quality of life of the patient in the bed than you have as a doctor. I think we have great problems in doing it without this input from the nurses. (DIM)

There is too much feeling. There is too much: oh, I am so sorry for this patient. No, they lack the comprehensive view, that there are 1,500 outside the door who are worse off than this patient. [...] My opinion is that when you are in the ward close to the patient you get a very good and valuable relation to this patient, but you miss the general view, where economy, other patients, and the need for the bed this patient is occupying now figure. [...] But you miss this comprehensive view when you are very close to a patient. (DSM)

There is at least one thing that I have heard very often, and that is that it is 'a pity for this patient', and that is a remark that has always irritated me. There is not much which is a pity for someone in that sense. What does it mean to be a pity for some other person. If you look into it, it is perhaps an expression of a lack of professional knowledge about the problem, and you need the professional knowledge to say something about the prognosis. Something can look hopeless and terrible and then it very quickly becomes a pity for the patient, but if you have a little more professional knowledge you can see that there is a chance that she will come out of it all right, so it

*is reasonable to continue. So maybe the differences are based in dif-
ferences in professional knowledge, I think that is the case.* (DSM)

On the other hand, nurses perceive some doctors as having too
little emotional contact with the patients:

> *I think that there is a tendency to – I don't now how much this has
> to do with ethics – to reify the issues. Look for instance at the somatic
> wards where the nurses perhaps focus more on the whole patient,
> because they are in contact with the patient all the time. But the
> doctor might come on a ward round with 5 minutes for each patient,
> and obviously has not … asks about the wound, the healing, the oper-
> ation, but may not hear that Mr. Hansen actually asks what was the
> result, expects that that has been given to you earlier, so I don't have
> to tell it again, and some doctors even get angry. They don't think it
> is their responsibility. […] In a somatic ward the doctors don't have
> much time for the individual patient, but the nurses do, we are on the
> ward.* (NIF)

The two different evaluations of the perceived difference
in ethical approach between nurses and doctors that are prevalent among physicians seem partially to determine how much
influence the physicians believe that nurses ought to have on
clinical decisions involving ethical problems. Most physicians
state that nurses should have a large say in such decisions. A
few disagree and claim that although nurses should be heard,
their influence on the decision should be restricted because
final responsibility rest with the physician. This second attitude is, in most cases, connected with the attitude that nurses
let their emotions play too prominent a role in their ethical
deliberations:

> *You obviously have to have the support of the other doctors. You
> should not act as an emperor, but these hyperdemocratic procedures
> that you – I once experienced at the department of neurology {…}
> where the cleaners where involved in discussing whether this or that
> patient should have this or that treatment, and there I think that we
> are far out. It has to be the professionals who have the courage, the
> knowledge, and the ability to make the necessary decisions. You can
> inform the other ranks, but I definitely do not think that an emotional
> assistant nurse should be able to influence a professional decision, de-
> finitely not.* (DSM)

A recent survey shows that of a random sample of internists 65 per cent believe that the nurses caring for a patient should participate in discussions about termination of treatment [24].

Apart from the fact that nurses usually spend more time with patients than doctors do, both groups give two other explanations for a possible difference in ethical approach. The first of these is the difference in emphasis on the medical/technical and the caring/non-technical aspects of health care in medical and nursing education. The second is the difference in final responsibility:

> *Nurses are often not conscious of the fact that it is physicians who have the final ethical responsibility. I mean, if we break some ethical laws, transgress some ethical limits, then we are held responsible. A nurse is never held responsible.* (DSM)

> *But I think that it is more difficult for the doctors, because they have to make the final decision. The nurses can put forward their opinions and thoughts, their input, what they have experienced with the patient, but the doctors have the final say.* (NIF)

Although the physician quoted here has an erroneous assessment of nurses' independent legal responsibility, it is nevertheless the case, as described above, that the final responsibility for making a decision will almost always fall on a physician. Even if a nurse refuses to carry out a prescription, the problem will revert to the physician, so it is only in cases where the decision of the nurse is either not to call a doctor, or in cases where a decision has to be made on the spot (e.g,. resuscitation decisions), that a nurse will have to take legal responsibility for the final decision.

Unfortunately, this legal situation does not solve nurses' ethical problems. In a situation where there is no legal reason to refuse to carry out a decision made by a physician, but where the nurse still believes that the decision is ethically problematic the ethical problem does not disappear if the nurse decides to 'follow orders'. Following an order that one believes to be ethically problematic, does not remove moral culpability, and may be followed by some kind of protest (see p. 191).

Philosophical attempts to solve this problem through

applications of Joseph Raz's arguments about second order reasoning has not resolved this problem satisfactorily [38–40]. Although the physician's training and (in most cases) better technical knowledge provide the nurse with a second order reason to follow the physician's orders, this second order reason can never be totally pre-emptive.

Should the structure of health care be changed?

The analysis in this chapter has pointed to several organisational features of the health care system that make a proper resolution of ethical problems difficult. It is evident that the main task of the health care system and the main duty of health care professionals are not the resolution of ethical problems. The main task is to help people who are ill or disabled. In the design of the organisation there must therefore be a balancing between the organisation best suited for the main task, and the organisation best suited for resolving ethical problems. What I want to suggest in the following is therefore not a total restructuring of the health care system, but some minor modifications which could possibly lead to a more satisfactory resolution of ethical problems. The two most important organisational factors which should be modified are: the external pressure causing time constraints, and the negative effects of hierarchical structures.

I cannot offer any immediate solutions to the first of these problems. There is at present a shortage of both nurses and doctors in Denmark, and when this is combined with a pressure to reduce waiting lists for operations, and a more general pressure to contain costs, it is difficult to believe that the situation will get better in the near future.

There are possible solutions to the second cluster of problems which contain two main subproblems. The first of these is that people low down in the hierarchy feel reticent about discussing ethical problems with their superiors, either because they feel that these superiors are not of a 'sufficient ethical standard', or because they are simply afraid of 'going out on a limb' and putting their job at risk by expressing divergent opinions. The second is that unethical behaviour by people high up in the hierarchy is not controlled very efficiently.

Both these subproblems could be addressed by introducing specific ethics conferences with the participation of independent ethics consultants. What I am suggesting is not the American model, with an ethicist on call ready to give advice at the bedside [41], but a regular discussion forum at which ethical problems can be brought up, and where somebody outside the hierarchical structure can act as a 'devil's advocate'. The ethics consultant can ask the awkward questions that insiders cannot ask, and give voice to disagreements that are otherwise not articulated. A successful realisation of this role would depend both on the ethics consultant having a formally recognised status within the organisation, and on the ethics consultant's personal skills.

Ethical problems in health care are of many different kinds, but a significant part of them can be grouped together in larger clusters (e.g., truth-telling, termination of treatment, the role of families in decision-making etc.). It is possible to develop fairly specific policies for problems in these clusters, detailing exactly what factors have to be taken into account in an ethical evaluation. Formal ethics conferences could aid the process of policy formulation, as well as having an important educational role.

It is important that both doctors and nurses participate in the ethics conference. Any discussion of policy should involve both professions, and the simple exercise of talking together about ethical problems in a neutral environment may change the common perception of differences between the ethical outlook of the two professions, or at least show that both perspectives are important for good ethical decision-making. Whether formal ethics conferences of the kind outlined here can work in the health care system, where traditionally the use of non-medical consultants has been minimal, is a question that can only be answered by further research.

Another possibility could be to introduce a similar figure to that of the patient adviser/advocate, which many hospitals are now introducing. If junior doctors and nurses had a doctors'/nurses' adviser with whom they could speak about 'unethical' superiors, and who could investigate such allegations, it could presumably help in identifying superiors of this type. It is, however, likely that such a person could not work effectively in an organisation of the size of the average hospital, since the identity of the complainant would often be easy to discover.

Notes

1 In the next sections I will refer to all discussions between professionals as conferences, even in those cases where they only involve two people.

References

1 Pugh, D. S., Hickson, D. J., *Writers on Organizations* (4th edn). London: Penguin Books, 1989.

2 Lundquist, L., *Byråkratisk etik*. Lund: Studentlitteratur, 1988.

3 Freidson, E., *Profession of Medicine – A Study of the Sociology of Applied Knowledge* (new edn). Chicago: University of Chicago Press, 1988.

4 Turner, B. S., *Medical Power and Social Knowledge*. London: Sage Publications, 1987.

5 Bakka, J. F., Fivelsdal, E., *Organisationsteori – Struktur, kultur, processer* (2. udg.). København: Handelshøjskolens Forlag, 1992.

6 Rydholm, I-M., *Att leda vård*. Göteborg: Nordiska Hälsovårdshögskolan, 1992.

7 Eriksen, E-O., Larsen, M-L., Ledelse og profesjonalitet. *Tidsskrift for den Norske Lægeforening* 1992; 112(14): 1855–9.

8 Bjørnsson, K., Kun læger har ordinationsret. *Sygeplejersken* 1995; 95(24): 22–5.

9 Sørensen, K., Groot, M-L., Jensen, H., Olsen, G., Sygeplejersker overskrider kompetence. *Sygeplejersken* 1995; 95(24): 8–11.

10 Turner, B. S., Knowledge, skill and occupational strategies: the professionalisation of paramedical groups. *Community Health Studies* 1985; 9: 38–47.

11 Simon, H. A., *Administrative Behavior* (3rd edn). New York: The Free Press, 1976.

12 March, J. G., Olsen, J. P., *Ambiguity and Choice in Organizations*. Bergen: Universitetsforlaget, 1976.

13 Lundquist, L., Ledarskapet och följarna. *Statsvetenskaplig Tidskrift* 1989; xx: 149–70.

14 Eriksen, H., Ulrichsen, H., *Tre kulturer i hospitalssektoren*. København: Nyt Nordisk Forlag, 1991.

15 Hofstede, G., *Culture's Consequences*. Newbury Park, CA: Sage Publica-

tions, 1980.

16 Borgenhammer, E., *Konvoj- eller lokomotivorganisation?* Lecture manuscript. Nordiska Hälsovårdshögskolan, 1992.

17 Borum, F., *Organisation, magt og forandring.* København: Nyt Nordisk Forlag, 1976.

18 Mechanic, D., *Medical Sociology* (2nd edn). New York: The Free Press, 1978.

19 Gardell, B., Gustafson, R. Å., *Sjukvård på löpande band.* Stockholm: Prisma, 1979.

20 Launsø, L., Jensen, H. M., *Sundhedsarbejde på tværs.* København: FADL's Forlag, 1980.

21 Atkinson, P., *Medical Talk and Medical Work.* London: Sage Publications, 1995.

22 White, B. D., Hickson, G. B., Theriot, R., Zaner, R. M., A medical ethics issues survey of residents in five pediatric training programs. *American Journal of the Diseases of Children* 1991; 145: 161–64.

23 Anspach, R., Notes on the sociology of medical discourse: the language of case presentation. *Journal of Health and Social Behavior* 1988; 29: 357–75.

24 Holm, S., The medical hierarchy and perceived influence on technical and ethical decisions. *Journal of Internal Medicine* 1995; 237: 487–92.

25 Howell, J. M,, Avolio, B. J., The ethics of charismatic leadership: submission or liberation. *Academy of Management Executive* 1992; 6(2): 43–54.

26 Seeman, M., Evans, J. W., Stratification and hospital care: 1. The performance of the medical intern. *American Sociological Review* 1961; 26(February): 67–80.

27 Seeman, M., Evans, J. W., Stratification and hospital care: 2. The objective criteria of performance. *American Sociological Review* 1961: 26(April): 193–204.

28 Sheehan, K. H., Sheehan, D. V., White, K., Leibowitz, A., Baldwin, D. C., A pilot study of medical student 'abuse' – student perceptions of mistreatment and misconduct in medical school. *JAMA* 1990; 263(4): 533–7.

29 Victor, B., Cullen, J. B., The organizational bases of ethical work climates. *Administrative Science Quarterly* 1988; 33(1): 101–25.

30 Hirschman, A. O., *Exit, Voice and Loyalty: Responses to Decline in Firms, Organizations and States.* Cambridge, MA: Harvard University Press, 1970.

31 Wall, A., *Ethics and the Health Services Manager.* London: King Edward's Hospital Fund for London, 1989.

32 French, P. A., *Ethics in Government.* Englewood Cliffs, NJ: Prentice-Hall Publishers, 1983.

33 Bok, S., *Secrets – On the Ethics of Concealment and Revelation.* New York: Vintage Books, 1989.

34 Bosk, C. L., *Forgive and Remember – Managing Medical Failure.*Chicago: University of Chicago Press, 1979.

35 Tschudin, V., Marks-Maran, D., *A Primer for Nurses – Workbook Ethics.* London: Baillière Tindall, 1993.

36 Anspach, R., Prognostic conflict in life-and-death decisions: the organization as an ecology of knowledge. *Journal of Health and Social Behavior*

1987; 28: 215–31.
37 Slomka, J., The negotiation of death: clinical decision-making at the end of life. *Social Science and Medicine* 1992; 35: 251–9.
38 May, T., The nurse under physician authority. *Journal of Medical Ethics* 1993; 19: 223–7.
39 Raz, J., *Practical Reasoning*. Oxford: Oxford University Press, 1978.
40 de Raeve, L., The nurse under physician authority: commentary. *Journal of Medical Ethics* 1993; 19: 228–9.
41 La Puma, J., Schiedermayer, D., *Ethics Consultation – A Practical Guide*. Boston: Jones and Bartlett Publishers, 1994.

6

From description to action

I do not think that there is any one non-ethical characteristic which is common and peculiar to everything that is intrinsically good. Nor do I think that all the self-evident principles of ethics can be brought under any one supreme principle. All attempts to do this seem quite plainly to over-simplify the actual situation. [1, pp. 283–4]

What use can be made of the account of the ethical perception and ethical reasoning of health care personnel which has been presented here so far? This final chapter will discuss two aspects of this question under the headings of generalisability and importance for normative ethics. In this way I will try to connect the findings to the theoretical argument presented in the first three chapters.

Can the description be generalised?

Because this is a qualitative study many medically trained researchers may want to raise a question such as the following: 'OK, you have described how your forty-two respondents think about ethical matters, and we may even grant you that the description seems to be thorough and meticulous, but how can you generalise from such a small non-random sample?'

The first response to this question must be to ask what is meant by 'generalise'. The simplest quantitative case is one in which we want to generalise from a sample to the population from which the sample was taken. In this case statistical sampling theory gives us tools with which we can estimate the margin of error for our generalisation. The more interesting case is the one in which we want to generalise from one population to another. When, for instance, we read that drug X is effective in the treatment of AIDS in American males, we want to generalise to our own country.

There is no doubt that if 'generalise' in the trans-population context means 'transfer quantitative results from one population to another', very few of the results of the present study can be generalised. There are very few quantitative results, and those there are are 'tainted' by the non-representative nature of the sampling of the respondents. If, however, 'generalise' means 'transfer knowledge to other settings' then a great proportion of the results can be generalised.

Whatever view we take on generalisation, between populations or across contexts, it is always the case that an argument is necessary before a generalisation can be claimed to be valid. This is the argument which should show that the situation we generalise from is similar in the relevant respects to the situation we wish to generalise to. In the medical context this argument is often not explicitly made, but only consists of an implied assumption about the uniform nature of human biology. That even this assumption is dubious in some circumstances can be illustrated by a simple quantitative example. Let us imagine that we have a methodologically perfect study showing that there is a strong inverse linear correlation between a woman's body-mass index and her tendency to develop osteoporosis, and that this study has been performed on the east coast of the USA. No matter how well the study had been performed, we could not generalise the findings to Bangladeshi women without first arguing that the large differences in wealth and nutritional status played no role with regard to this correlation.

Similarly, generalisation from a qualitative study depends on arguing that such generalisation is valid. What we cannot generalise from qualitative studies are numbers, frequencies, and numerical correlations. What we can generalise are expla-

nations, structures, and frameworks. In a paper on the methodology of case-studies Stake notes that it is really possible to
obtain general knowledge, even from individual cases:

> From case reports we learn both propositional and experiential
> knowledge [...]. Certain descriptions and assertions are assimilated
> by readers into memory. When the researcher's narrative provides
> opportunity for vicarious experience, readers extend their memo-
> ries of happenings.
>
> [...]
>
> The reader comes to know some things told, as if he or she had
> experienced them. Enduring meanings come from encounter, and
> are modified and reinforced by repeated encounter. [2, p. 240]

Some writers on qualitative methods believe that such a
transfer of concepts is not generalisation, and that qualitative
researchers should be content with providing thick descriptions. Zyzanski *et al.* thus write:

> The qualitative researcher is not particularly bothered by a lack of
> generalizability. He or she is under no illusion that his or her obser-
> vations and interpretations necessarily apply to other persons,
> events or contexts. Rather he or she endeavors to construct as thick
> and detailed a description as possible of his or her particular set-
> ting and circumstances so that others who encounter his or her
> description can determine its possible applicability to their setting
> and circumstances. While epidemiology seeks the logic of general-
> izability, qualitative research acknowledges the possibility of con-
> cept applicability or transferability but makes no claim that it
> necesarily occurs. [3, p. 245]

To me, it seems that this quote contains a profound contradiction. It may well be true that the qualitative researcher is not
particularly bothered if her or his findings cannot be generalised to *all* remotely similar contexts, but the qualitative
researcher who is not bothered if her or his findings cannot be
generalised to *any* even closely similar context must be a very
strange kind of researcher. If research aims at producing something more than a literary work in the genre 'research report',
it must aim at some kind of generalisability. Zyzanski *et al.* are
correct in emphasising that generalisations are never necessarily

valid, but every research project must endeavour to reach a stage where generalisations are at least possible.

In what follows I will therefore try to outline answers to two questions; to what extent can the findings about ethical perception and reasoning be generalised to health care professionals outside Denmark? and to what extent can the findings on the influence of the health care organisation be generalised? These two questions are closely related, and an answer to the first will also be a partial answer to the second.

Problems in generalisation

The possibility of valid generalisation of the ethical framework to other countries will mainly depend on the extent to which the socialisation and working conditions of the non-Danish population of health care professionals are different from those of the population studied here. With regard to the socialisation of health care professionals Danish medical schools are characterised by a substantially lower level of work pressure than medical schools in the USA and Britain, and by a substantially higher student influence on various aspects of medical education. Through a lower 'selection pressure' this could lead to a less 'elitist' socialisation, which could affect the possibility of generalisation.

In the organisation of health care, there are probably at least three factors that are important. At the level of organisational structure the relative paucity of explicit rules referring certain decisions to specific levels in the hierarchy is probably important for the relative uniformity of ethical outlook found in Denmark. In systems where status differences in the hierarchy are more clearly marked, greater differences could be seen.

The distance in social status and power between doctors and nurses in Denmark is relatively small, and this is probably important for the degree of similarity between the respondents in the present study. In countries that are similar to Denmark in other ways, but where there is greater social distance between the roles of doctors and nurses, it is likely that the ethical framework of the two professions will diverge more. Given the fact that nurses are often female and doctors often male, it is also likely that their ethical frameworks may diverge more in cultures where gender differences are emphasised more than in Denmark.

Finally, Denmark has a public health care system with equal access and free treatment for all citizens. This structural feature is likely to influence the ethical framework. Justice issues are, for instance, not as acute as in a system where many people are without access to health care – in Denmark those who use the health care system use it as users and citizens, and not as consumers. These considerations indicate that a generalisation to an American population of health care professionals would be much more likely to be wrong than a generalisation to a British or a German context.

Danish health care professionals are almost all salaried employees, and are not providing fee-for-service medicine. Some conflicts of interests which are prominent in other arrangements thereby disappear, and others appear. A generalisation is therefore most likely to be valid if it is in a context where health care professionals are also salaried employees.

With regard to the influence of organisational features on the ethical framework, the alternative actions identified can probably be generalised fairly widely, but the exact way in which they are used will depend on the specific structural features of the given health care system. In systems with larger status differences, and more strict control of the performance of subordinates, the visible forms of protest may, for instance, be suppressed.

Thick description and normative ethics

As I already pointed out in Chapter 4, the ethical framework of health care professionals does not conform to any of the classical theories of ethics. It is therefore relevant to assess what implication this finding – and the findings on ethical perception and the influence of the organisation – could have for normative ethics.

There is no doubt that the fact that health care professionals presently have a specific ethical framework has no normative implications in itself. Their ethical framework could have been evil through and through and in need of radical reconstruction. The content and structure of the framework could, however, have some implications when we consider how we can change or modify the ethical behaviour of health care professionals through education. New principles which can fit the framework without changing the structure will presumably be easier to adopt than new principles which require major structural change. This argument could therefore suggest that the best approach to ethical education of health care professionals is aimed at incremental improvement and not radical change.

But is this not also an irrelevant consideration seen from a normative point of view? Why should we worry about whether it is easy or difficult for health care professionals to adopt our principles? The only thing that matters is whether these principles are the right principles.

Whether this is a cogent objection depends on what the purpose of normative ethics is. Within a consequentialist theory it could, for instance, make sense to try to get a 'second best' principle adopted, if this would lead to better consequences in the long run than an attempt to get 'the best' principle adopted (e.g., because it was very difficult).

This brings us back to the discussion of acceptance, conformance, and pluralistic utility in Chapter 2. It is by now almost a platitude that we live in a pluralistic society, but it is (unfortunately?) a true platitude, at least in the sense that very few societies are totally homogeneous. This means that our normative ethical guidelines have to be functional in a setting where there is a plurality of different ethical frameworks. The findings in the present study may make it a little easier to 'calculate' how other agents in the health care setting will act, in response to the promulgation of a specific rule, or just in response to actions I perform. In this way the findings are of normative interest, both at a strategic level of detached normative thinking, and at the everyday tactical level of ethical decision-making.

With regard to education there might also be a case for emphasising ethical perception skills, instead of ethical theory or ethical reasoning skills. The most prominent differences between health care professionals found in this study are differences in what they perceive as ethical problems. When they have realised that they have an ethical problem, most are able to put forward very reasonable ethical arguments. Developing educational measures which enhance ethical perception may therefore be a relatively simple way to enhance ethical decision-making.

Better ethics or better organisation?

The findings about the influence of the organisation on ethical perception and ethical reasoning should also possibly lead to a redirection of some of our efforts in normative medical ethics. If it is really true that organisational structures and key persons in the organisation have a large influence on ethical decisions, which in some cases overrides the ethical reasoning of individual health care professionals, then it might be prudent to direct more attention to the question of how we can build 'ethical organisations'.

Within the management literature it is possible to find studies that look at this issue but there are also large areas of neglect. Many of the eighteen research propositions about the connection between organisation and ethics that Trevino put forward in 1986 have not yet been researched [4], and even more of them have not been researched in the context of health care organisations.

In the end, the practical goal of medical ethics must be more ethical treatment of patients, and if this goal is more easily reached by organisational change than by changing the personal ethics of health care professionals, then ethicists should perhaps take more interest in organisational theory and in the dynamics of organisational change. Exactly how an organisation should be structured in order to promote ethical behaviour is not immediately obvious, and the answer to that question probably requires a mix of both theoretical reflection and empirical study.

Simplification or realism

It is a consistent feature of most ethical theory that it tries to subsume all ethical judgement under one specific theoretical idea (maximisation of consequences, reverence for moral law, etc.). This is understandable given the emphasis on consistency and simplicity which guides philosophical reflection in the analytic tradition.

The ethical framework of health care professionals is obviously different. It incorporates a number of, at least potentially, contradictory considerations. This difference could perhaps in a contemplative moment lead one to ponder whether Ockham's razor should be used as aggressively in ethics as in other parts of philosophy. Do we really have strong reasons to believe that a simple ethical theory is better in the requisite sense than a complicated theory?

An adequate answer to this question requires a much longer discussion than I am able to present here. I do, however, think that it is worth noting that most 'single idea' theories in ethics only reach their unifying goal by redescribing other moral considerations in a way that distorts the commonsense understanding of their function. It may be that consequences, rights, and virtues are really different things which are not reducible to each other, and which are all important for moral theory.

References

1 Broad, C. D., *Five Types of Ethical Theory*. London: Routledge and Kegan Paul, 1930.

2 Stake, R. E., Case studies. In: Denzin, N. K., Lincoln, Y. S. (eds), *Handbook of Qualitative Research*. Thousand Oaks, CA: Sage Publications, 1994: pp. 236–47.

3 Zyzanski, S. J., McWhinney, I. R., Blake, R., Crabtree, B. F., Miller, W. L., Qualitative research: perspectives on the future. In: Crabtree, B. F., Miller, W. L. (eds), *Doing Qualitative Research*. Newbury Park, CA: Sage Publications, 1992: pp. 231–48.

4 Trevino, L. K., Ethical decision making in organizations: a person–situation interactionist model. *Academy of Management Review* 1986; 11(3): 601–17.

Sonnet — To Science

Science! true daughter of Old Time thou art!
Who alterest all things with thy peering eyes.
Why preyest thou thus upon the poet's heart,
Vulture, whose wings are dull realities?
How should he love thee? or how deem thee wise,
Who wouldst not leave him in his wandering
To seek for treasure in the jewelled skies,
Albeit he soared with an undaunted wing?
Hast thou not dragged Diana from her car?
And driven the Hamadryad from the wood
To seek a shelter in some happier star?
Hast thou not torn the Naiad from her flood,
The Elfin from the green grass, and from me
The summer dream beneath the tamarind tree?

Edgar Allan Poe. *The Raven and Other Favorite Poems*. New York: Dover Publications, 1991 (original 1845): p. 8.

Index